CONTENTS

LIST OF FIGURES

LIST OF TABLES

Report of a Working Party of the Standing Medical Advisory Committee on Sickle Cell, Thalassaemia and other Haemoglobinopathies

POLICY IN CONFIDENCE

London: HMSO

INTRODUCTION

I welcome the publication of this report and heartily endorse its recommendations which should prove helpful for purchasers of health care and providers of treatment. Moreover, I believe the implementation of the recommendations will provide a comprehensive service which will benefit enormously the families and communities affected by sickle cell anaemia and other haemoglobinopathies.

Cumberlege.

BARONESS CUMBERLEGE

ISBN 0 11 321699 8

Members of the Working Party

Professor Alan G Johnson MChir, FRCS (Chairman)
Professor of Surgery
University of Sheffield

Dr Elizabeth N Anionwu RGN, HV Tutor, PhD
Lecturer in Community Genetic Counselling
Unit of Clinical Genetics and Fetal Medicine
Institute of Child Health, London

Ms Merry France-Dawson RMN, RGN, MA
Freelance Researcher
Nominated by the Royal College of Nursing
20 Cavendish Square, London

Dr Milica Brozovic MD, FRCPath
Consultant Haematologist
Central Middlesex HospitalNHS Trust, London, NW10 7NS

Professor CJ Dickinson DM, FRCP
Consultant Physician and Emeritus Professor of Medicine
Wolfson Institute of Preventive Medicine
St Bartholemew's Hospital Medical College
Charterhouse Square, London

Mr Stephen AD Miles MB, BCh, FRCSEd
Consultant in Accident and Emergency Medicine
St. Bartholemew's Hospital
West Smithfield, London, EC1A 7BE
Honorary Secretary and nominated by British Association for Accident and Emergency Medicine
Also, Royal College of Surgeons of England
35 – 43 Lincoln's Inn Fields, London, WC2A 3PN

Professor A Bellingham FRCP, FRCPath
Consultant Haematologist,
Department of Haematological Medicine
King's College School of Medicine and Dentistry
Denmark Hill, London

Dr Anita Holdcroft MD, FRCA
Senior Lecturer and Honorary Consultant Anaesthetist,
Department of Anaesthetics
Hammersmith Hospital
Du Cane Hospital, London W12 0NN

Dr Bernadette Modell FRCP, FRC Path
Wellcome Principal Research Fellow in Community Genetics,
Department of Obstetrics and Gynaecology
University College London Medical School
86 – 96 Chenies Mews, London, WC1E 6HX

Mr K Charalampous AAT
The Thalassaemia Society
107 NIghtingale Lane, London, N8

Dr R Milne BA, MSc, MFPHM
Consultant in Public Health Medicine,
Oxford Regional Health Authority
Old Road
Headington
Oxford

Dr R MacFaul MB, ChB, FRCP
Consultant Paediatrician,
Wakefield HA
Pinderfields General Hospital
Aberford Road
Wakefield
West Yorkshire

Dr Ivan G Cox FRCGP, MRCP, DCH
General Practitioner,
Laurie Pike Health Centre
95 Birchfield Road
Handsworth
Birmingham

Ms Cecilia Olojo
Sickle Cell Housing Officer
Organisation for Sickle Cell Anaemia Research

Ms S Edwards (Died 26th November 1992)

Dr A Rejman, (Medical Secretariat) MD, MRCP, MRCPath
Senior Medical Officer
Department of Health

Miss T A Dighton (Administrative Secretariat) BSc
Department of Health

Mrs V Keating (Administrative Sectretariat) BSc, MSc
Formerly Department of Health

FOREWORD

The inherited disorders of Haemoglobin – Sickle Cell Disorder and Thalassaemia, in particular present difficult challenges to Health Authorities and those professionals providing care and advice to families and patients whether demographic factors result in a high or low prevalence.

The disorders vary in clinical severity, yet prophylactic medicine, knowledge of the condition, proper crisis intervention and expert management can alleviate complications.

The Standing Medical Advisory Committee welcomed the opportunity to address these issues and to offer advice to the Secretaries of State for Health and Wales. It is indebted to the Working Party, chaired by Professor Alan Johnson, for an excellent and comprehensive report.

SMAC considers that the report is a helpful basis for those who are responsible for defining provision for patients and families at risk from these disorders. It should enable achievement of the best possible care and will provide a focus for further debate, development and collaboration.

Dr Nuala Sterling CBE, FRCP

Chairman SMAC

SMAC WORKING PARTY ON SICKLE CELL, THALASSAEMIA AND OTHER HAEMOGLOBINOPATHIES

EXECUTIVE SUMMARY

The Secretary of State for Health invited the Standing Medical Advisory Committee (SMAC) to consider various aspects of haemoglobinopathies, in order to ensure more even provision of health care.

The haemoglobinopathies are an inherited group of disorders of varying clinical severity with potentially serious and crippling complications. Prophylactic medicine, knowledge of the condition, proper crisis intervention and expert management can alleviate the complications.

Screening enables patients and doctors to be alert to the disorders and potential parents to make informed choices in pregnancy.

This working party has sparked a tremendous amount of interest, from health professionals (both individuals and professional bodies), people with haemoglobinopathies and their families, members of populations at risk and relevant voluntary organisations. This concern was reflected by the large number of people and organisations who submitted written evidence.

All the Regional Health Authorities provided details on the provision of services for people with haemoglobinopathies and populations at risk in Districts within their Regions. Voluntary organisations also commented on provision of services, often with particular reference to problems encountered by people with sickle cell disorder (SCD) and thalassaemia.

It was clear from both oral and written evidence that care for patients with haemoglobinopathies, and genetic counselling of populations at risk, is not always of the highest quality, even where these disorders are frequently seen.

Recommendations have been made which allow responses by specific groups who may need to act upon them. These groups are: purchasers of health care; those responsible for clinical management, counselling and screening services; Government agencies and Departments; medical educational bodies; general practitioners and other providers of treatment; patients and patient groups.

If the recommendations are followed then patients, families and whole communities will receive the type of comprehensive care from which they should benefit.

The importance of these disorders was brought home forcefully in November 1992 when Sharon Edwards, the working party's original patient representative for SCD, died as a result of her condition. It is hoped that this report and the consequent improvement of services for patients with haemoglobinopathies will be a fitting memorial to her.

SECTION 1 • INTRODUCTION

"We try to achieve as much as we can, we try to get ahead, and when we have setbacks like losing a job it really is a let down. Some people do have difficulty in coming to terms with this and they really do need a lot of encouragement and they need a lot of push; you can achieve so much. One day I just got up and said "Right, that's it, enough is enough, I'm going to fight you". It's a matter of whether you control the sickle cell or the sickle cell will control you. You can't let it get to you, get you down. I know it is very difficult because I am going through it – but you can achieve a lot.' Sharon Edwards (*Ref 1*)

THE WORKING PARTY

PURPOSE

The Secretary of State for Health invited the Standing Medical Advisory Committee (SMAC) to consider various aspects of haemoglobinopathies, in order to ensure more even provision of health care. SMAC, therefore, set up a Working Party, which was chaired by Professor A G Johnson. Members of the Working Party are listed on pages 5 – 6.

The haemoglobinopathies are an inherited group of disorders of varying clinical severity with potentially serious and crippling complications. Prophylactic medicine, knowledge of the condition, proper crisis intervention and expert management can alleviate the complications.

Screening enables patients and doctors to be alert to the disorders and potential parents to make informed choices in pregnancy.

There was evidence that **such patients are not always looked after in the best possible way, even in districts where these disorders are common**. In addition, many patients come from already disadvantaged minorities. Thus purchasers (acting on behalf of patients) and providers need to take these concerns into consideration.

TERMS OF REFERENCE

To consider issues relating to the screening, counselling, and clinical management of people affected by sickle cell disorder, thalassaemia and other haemoglobinopathies; to advise on the information which should be provided about the haemoglobinopathies to those affected and to health professionals and to give advice on the assessment of need, provision of facilities, treatment and measurement of outcomes.

The working party primarily considered SCD and thalassaemia and not Homozygous Haemoglobin C (HbCC), Homozygous Haemoglobin D (HbDD) and others with few clinical problems. There are numerous other haemoglobinopathies manifesting themselves clinically in different ways. These are rare conditions and are not related to any specific ethnic group. The majority of these conditions are relatively benign and are not associated with clinical and social problems.

SMAC has a statutory duty to advise the Secretaries of State for Health and Wales on medical matters. However, data has necessarily been included for other parts of the UK. The working party has been in contact with the Scottish Home and Health Department (SHHD) and Northern Ireland Office who will receive copies of the report.

METHOD OF WORKING

Groups and individuals with an interest – patient groups, professional carers, purchasers and providers – were asked for evidence and were represented on the Working Party. Details of individuals and groups who submitted evidence is in Appendix 1. Representations were made in both written and oral evidence, by patients and patient organisations requesting that the Department of Health consider free prescriptions for people with haemoglobinopathies. **The setting up of the Working Party sparked widespread interest, especially among patient groups.** An example of comments highlighted by one body is in Appendix 2.

As the report necessarily includes some technical terms readers are referred to the glossary. For ease of reading where appropriate the masculine 'he' should be taken to also cover the feminine 'she'.

DEFINITIONS

Sickle cell disorder (SCD) and **thalassaemia** are autosomal recessive inherited disorders **(Figure 2, Appendix 3) affecting the structure or synthesis of haemoglobin**, the red pigment principally responsible for the carriage of oxygen by the red cells of the blood .

It is essential to make a clear distinction between **carriers** who carry a haemoglobinopathy trait, who are very numerous and the much smaller number of people with the disorders. In different ethnic groups at risk, from 1 in 30 to 1 in 4 of the whole population are carriers. They are perfectly healthy, but can be identified by simple blood tests. However, they have a genetic risk. If a carrier chooses a non-carrier partner, in each pregnancy there is a 1 in 2 chance that the child will be a carrier but **no risk** of him having the disorder, and the condition is often transmitted in this way through many generations without causing health problems. However, if **both** partners are carriers, in each pregnancy there is a 1 in 4 risk that the child may inherit an abnormal haemoglobin gene from **both** parents, and the child is likely to have a major haemoglobin disorder. Depending on ethnic group, at birth there are from 17 to 100 times as many carriers as affected children. – See Table 1 below.

TABLE 1: EXAMPLES OF FREQUENCIES OF HAEMOGLOBIN TRAITS (CARRIERS) IN CERTAIN ETHNIC GROUPS

Haemoglobin Type	Ethnic Group	Carrier Frequency
Sickle Cell Trait	Afro-Caribbeans	1 in 10
	West Africans	up to 1 in 4
	Cypriots	1 in 100
	Pakistanis, Indians	1 in 100
C Trait	Afro-Caribbeans	1 in 30
	Ghanaians	up to 1 in 6
D Trait	Indians, Pakistanis	1 in 100
	White British	1 in 1000
Alpha Thalassaemia	Chinese	1 in 15 – 1 in 30
	Cypriots	1 in 50 – 1 in 100
Beta Thalassaemia	Cypriots	1 in 7
	Asians	1 in 10 – 1 in 30
	Chinese	1 in 30
	Afro-Caribbeans	1 in 50
	White British	1 in 1000

NB. Not all ethnic groups are included. More details, including details about frequencies in other populations, can be obtained from Appendix 3.

There are about 5000 people with SCD in the UK, primarily in the Afro-Caribbean population. The term 'SCD' usually refers not only to homozygous sickle cell anaemia (SS) but also to sickle cell/ haemoglobin C disease (SC) and sickle/beta thalassaemia.

In **SCD** the red cells change from a round to a sickle shape when the amount of oxygen in the blood is decreased. Much of the treatment of patients with SCD relates to acute, unpredictable events. The typical picture of SCD in patients in the UK is of repeated painful crises when the sickled cells become trapped in small blood vessels. These require analgesia and rehydration as well as treatment of infection which may precipitate the crises.

The severity, duration and frequency of crises is variable between patients and sometimes may change during the lifetime of an individual patient. Other important clinical episodes may include aplastic crises, where infection may cause the bone marrow to fail to produce red cells, strokes in children, and sequestration of red cells by the spleen. Management of pregnant patients with SCD require special considerations in addition to those for other individuals. Where general anaesthesia is required, the anaesthetist and surgeon need to know the diagnosis in order to take appropriate measures.

Thalassaemia, mostly of the 'beta' type, is less common and in homozygous form **affects about 600 people in the UK**. This population is mainly derived from the Mediterranean and Indian sub-continent. There is a much larger number of individuals who are heterozygotes and have haemoglobinopathy traits as mentioned above (see Appendix 3 and Table 1). Alpha zero thalassaemia is rare and affects mainly people of South East Asian (Chinese) origin.

Thalassaemia (named from the Greek for near the sea) differs from SCD in that the mainstay of treatment is predictable. Thalassaemia causes a failure to produce normal haemoglobin as well as increased breakdown of red cells. This leads to a severe anaemia and the body tries to increase production of red cells by increasing the marrow capacity in bones as well as increasing the size of the spleen and liver. The bones and spleen also increase in size to try to cope with the breakdown of red cells. Patients require regular blood transfusion, usually monthly, and continual chelation therapy to prevent excessive deposition of iron in the various organs of the body.

Both groups of haemoglobinopathy genes can also be divided into severe forms (that cause disease in the homozygous state) and mild ones (that cause disease only when combined with a severe form).

The **frequency** of haemoglobinopathy disorders in certain ethnic groups leads to a concentration of patients in some districts, many of which are in inner cities, often in deprived areas. Appropriate services may have to be provided in every District on occasion, e.g. for someone with a haemoglobinopathy taking a holiday in the area.

SELF-HELP GROUPS

There are numerous national and local self-help groups which represent the interests of patients with haemoglobinopathies and their families. **Associations such as the Sickle Cell Society, the Organisation for Sickle Cell Anaemia Research (OSCAR) and the UK Thalassaemia Society have an important role to play in increasing community awareness and promoting carrier screening.** They also provide invaluable help to counsellors in the form of posters, and information leaflets and booklets that can be given to members of communities at risk before screening, and where a carrier has been identified. They often provide a contact point for enquiries, and allow carriers and families of patients to meet each other.

OCCURRENCE OF HAEMOGLOBIN DISORDERS IN ENGLAND AND WALES

The occurrence of the haemoglobinopathies in the UK depends on the number and distribution of the ethnic groups at risk, and on the characteristics of their carrier states, marriage trends and birth rates. **The birth rate and the total numbers in each ethnic group are both relevant to service planning. In addition the effectiveness, acceptability and costs of intervention measures need to be considered when determining use of resources.**

NUMBERS OF ETHNIC MINORITIES

An estimate of the number and distribution of the main groups at risk can be derived from the 1991 census figures. However, even in the 1991 census, categorisation is not detailed enough to allow identification of some at risk groups such as Cypriots and Italians (see Section 3 for further information). The effect of population movements on the frequency of haemoglobinopathies in North West Europe has been studied in detail by the World Health Organisation (*Ref 2*).

The figures suggest that about 6% of the population of England and about 10% of all births are in groups at risk for haemoglobinopathy disorders (Appendix 3).

GEOGRAPHICAL DISTRIBUTION

The distribution of persons aged under 5 belonging to ethnic minority groups is summarised in Figure 1. Though ethnic minorities tend to be concentrated in the conurbations, **every NHS Region has at least one area with a significant number of births in relevant ethnic groups. Every Regional Director of Public Health therefore has a role in ensuring that purchasers demand the relevant carrier screening and appropriate counselling.**

BIRTH RATES

All but the longest-established ethnic groups have a young age-distribution (Figure 2), and thus a relatively high birth rate. Therefore, the need for screening and counselling will increase rather than decrease in the future. Some families have large numbers of children; but these numbers are falling fast among British Pakistanis and Bangladeshis as the new generation increasingly uses family planning and other services.

NUMBERS OF PEOPLE WITH HAEMOGLOBINOPATHY TRAITS

Most information on carrier rates is based on studies made in the countries of origin of the different groups, but the observed birth-rates of affected infants in the UK are consistent with the figures shown in Appendix 3. **There is tremendous variation in the haemoglobinopathy genes found in different ethnic groups, and no specific haemoglobinopathy is confined to a single ethnic group.**

MARRIAGE TRENDS

Expected annual births of affected children will also depend on marriage trends. Some groups (Afro-Caribbeans, Cypriots, Italians) frequently marry outside their ethnic group. **This obviously reduces the genetic risk for the next generation, but in the long-term dissociates risk from the ethnic group.** Other communities still largely marry within their own group. Pakistanis, and to a lesser extent Bangladeshis, have a positive tradition of marriage between closely-related individuals, which increases the chances of a couple conceiving an affected child (*Ref 3*).

MAIN HAEMOGLOBINOPATHIES

Table 2 below shows the main haemoglobinopathies causing SCD and thalassaemia in the UK. Unfortunately the International Classification of Disease:10 (ICD 10) does not give a detailed breakdown. An improved classification is currently being developed by a Haematology Working Party looking at Read Classification and Diagnostic Working Groups, which is likely to report by the end of 1993.

Table 2: The main haemoglobinopathies causing SCD and Thalassaemia in the UK – based on ICD 10 classification.

SICKLE CELL DISORDER

- Sickle cell anaemia (HbSS)
- Sickle cell beta thalassaemia
- Hb SC (Sickle Haemoglobin C Disease)
- Hb SD (Sickle Haemoglobin D Disease)
- Hb SE (Sickle Haemoglobin E disease)
- Other rare sickle-cell disorders

THALASSAEMIA

- Beta thalassaemia – major
- Beta thalassaemia – intermedia
- Hb E Beta thalassaemia
- Other rare forms of thalassaemia
- Alpha thalassaemia (Hb Barts hydrops fetalis)
- Hb H disease

Figure 1 : 1991 Census : Percentage of persons aged under 5 belonging to ethnic minority groups by local authority district

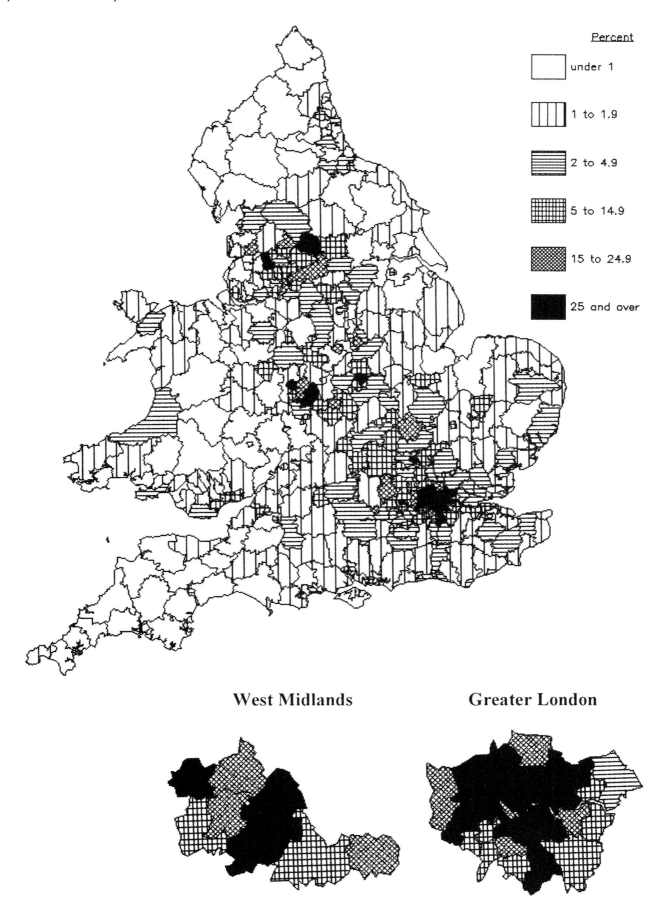

Percent

under 1

1 to 1.9

2 to 4.9

5 to 14.9

15 to 24.9

25 and over

West Midlands

Greater London

Produced by the Institute of Public Health, University of Surrey, March 1993

Figure 2 : Age distribution of some ethnic groups – England and Wales

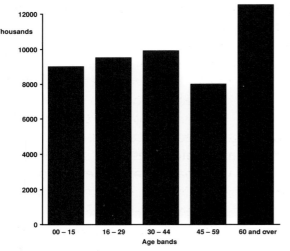

Table 1. White

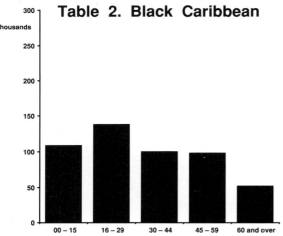

Table 2. Black Caribbean

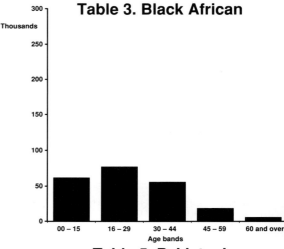

Table 3. Black African

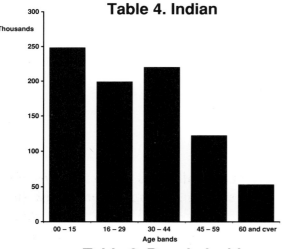

Table 4. Indian

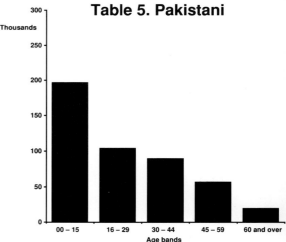

Table 5. Pakistani

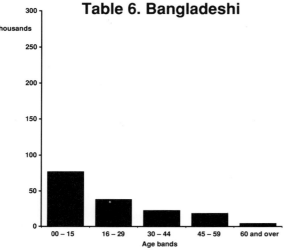

Table 6. Bangladeshi

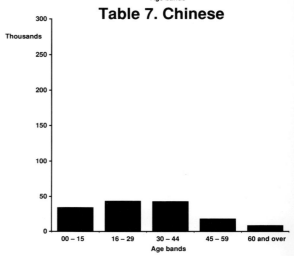

Table 7. Chinese

ETHNIC GROUPS

It is important to stress the difference between nationality and ethnicity. A suggested question that may be asked of pregnant women to determine whether to screen her for haemo-globinopathies can be something like the following: "Were you, or your partner's, parents or grandparents, on either side, born in the UK or Ireland?" or "Are you sure that all your ancestors were born in the UK or Ireland?". "If not where did they come from? Please indicate the name of the country, or point to it on the map provided." **It needs to be emphasised that this sort of questioning is not concerned with the right to domicile.** These questions also need to be asked about the father of the child. The Working Party discussions highlighted difficulties in a universally-applicable categorisation of ethnicity. The 1991 Census categories were considered deficient because the main ones did not indicate groups which were particularly relevant to thalassaemia, e.g. Greek and Turkish Cypriots, Italians or people of Middle Eastern origin. A more detailed and more helpful division is given by the Code Numbers in the OPCS 1991 Census Coding Frame (Ref 4). It is important to note that the **place of birth** of an individual may be totally different from his or her **ethnic background**. In 1992 the NHS Management Executive issued guidance on the collection of information on patients' ethnic group (*Ref 5*).

This information is relevant not only for those individuals having both parents and grandparents or other ancestors from these countries, but also for those who have only one parent, grandparent or other ancestor from these countries.

The following list is not comprehensive but provides information on the countries from which come people likely to be at risk, and who are present in significant numbers in the UK.

ASIA e.g.
India (including East African Asians)
Pakistan
Bangladesh
Sri Lanka

FAR EAST e.g.
China – Hong Kong
Malaysia
Thailand
Philippines
Vietnam

AFRICA

MIDDLE EAST e.g.
Saudi Arabia
Kuwait
Iran
Iraq
Qatar

MEDITERRANEAN e.g.
Cyprus
Greece
Turkey
Italy

CARIBBEAN e.g..
Jamaica
Trinidad
Barbados

OTHERS – all areas of the New World have substantial populations at risk of haemoglobinopathies whose ancestors have migrated from the above areas.

GENERAL CONCEPTS

Screening, applied discerningly, plays an essential part in offering choices to couples – to detect carrier status or presymptomatic states – thus allowing them options on how to proceed. If intervention gives benefit to the individuals concerned it may be appropriate to offer screening to populations, or to selected groups, families, couples and individuals at risk (*Ref 6*).

Decisions about whether or not screening is necessary depend on the severity, mortality and morbidity of a particular condition. The incidence and mode of inheritance, together with any risk to an individual of being tested, determines whether screening should be carried out universally or selectively. **Screening is only valuable if it influences action.** Possible interventions come under three main headings: education, counselling and treatment.

The incidence of a disorder in various racial, ethnic, religious or cultural groups within a population will also help determine screening policy; but due regard must be paid to the principles of fairness and justice. A screening programme must comply with the general principles of screening which have been discussed elsewhere (*Refs 7, 8*)

BENEFITS/DISADVANTAGES

The most obvious potential **benefit** for individuals is the **reassurance that they are <u>not</u> at risk**. For affected individuals, the advantage of early diagnosis and treatment are manifest in **prolonged survival and quality of life**. Possible benefits are effective therapy, removal of uncertainty, and better informed plans for occupation, finance and family. **Disadvantages** might be the **realisation that cure is not at present possible**, and fear, anxiety, a threatened future, loss of self-esteem, and difficulties with occupation and insurance. A further disadvantage, in the case of antenatal testing of the mother, is the **small risk to the fetus of antenatal diagnosis.** This is particularly relevant where the outcome of the test would not affect the mother's decision about whether or not to terminate the pregnancy.

OPPORTUNITIES FOR SCREENING

Screening may be performed at various stages in the life of an individual.
It may be carried out **preconceptionally** or **antenatally** to detect parents at risk of having an affected child. **Neonatal screening** is performed after birth to detect affected infants.

ADULT SCREENING

Opportunistic screening occurs when an adult patient at risk of SCD or has a blood test result suggesting that the individual may be a carrier, or presents with symptoms suggestive of disorder. When an individual at risk requires surgery, either planned or in an emergency. The individual must be screened for SCD unless the urgency of the situation dictates that the operation needs to start before the result is available.

Table 3 summarises the possible stages at which screening may be carried out and the objectives determining the programme. Technical details are available in the specialist literature (*Refs 9, 10*)

PRECONCEPTIONAL SCREENING

When screening is carried out only during pregnancy, people can find they have to make some very difficult decisions in undue haste and a distressed state. It is therefore recognised that **services should evolve towards preconceptional diagnosis and counselling. GPs have an important role to play here and may suggest such screening when patients first register at the practice.**

There are few GPs in the country who can claim that they have no families registered with them in ethnic groups at risk. They are in an excellent position to **check that women of reproductive age have been offered testing for haemoglobinopathies, before starting a pregnancy.** Such testing and advice could, for example, be included in family planning or preconceptional counselling clinics.

ANTENATAL SCREENING

Every child with a major haemoglobinopathy disorder has two parents who are carriers of the disorder. Therefore in theory every affected birth could be predicted by antenatal screening.

Figure 3 is a flow-chart of the way that antenatal screening should work. With an appropriate service all pregnant carriers of alpha or beta thalassaemia, or of a sickling gene or other haemoglobin variant (e.g. haemoglobin C or D), should be detected and informed. This is obviously impossible when testing is refused.

The decision on whether to do selective or universal screening can be difficult and is particularly pressing in the case of SCD. Table 3 gives guidelines which are easy to follow if the number of antenatal patients from ethnic groups at-risk are either very low or very high. If the population of the antenatal clinic includes more than 15% ethnic minorities at-risk of SCD there needs to be universal antenatal and neonatal screening. As already mentioned, the overall proportion of such ethnic groups in the general population in a district may not properly reflect the number of antenatal patients, if the age distribution and fertility is different for different ethnic groups. **Policy decisions must be made locally and be well-informed.**

If a decision is made to screen selectively, a policy must be determined locally on how to assess an individual's ethnic origin (see page 19 in Section 2). Clear instructions must be transmitted to those who carry out the policy — primarily midwives and GPs. This may have continuous training implications due to staff changes. Additionally all policies, whether universal or selective, must **include a protocol for informing women and their partners of the results of tests, whether positive or negative for a haemoglobinopathy gene. Counselling should be offered as appropriate.**

SICKLE CELL DISORDER

For SCD there was a relatively low uptake of antenatal diagnosis in the early years. The reasons for this have not been formally investigated but may include the following: (a) Initially only mid-trimester antenatal diagnosis was available, and was less acceptable for SCD than first trimester antenatal diagnosis; (b) Many doctors decided that antenatal diagnosis was not appropriate for SCD, because of the unpredictability of the disorder, though antenatal screening of mothers at risk is mandatory because of the maternal obstetric implications. Furthermore, there was no provision of information, counselling, or the offer of antenatal diagnosis; (c) It is difficult for couples to decide for or against antenatal diagnosis for SCD, owing to the inability to predict the severity and outcome of the disorder in the individual fetus. This needs expert counselling, which initially was not widely available. **Uptake of antenatal diagnosis for SCD increased with the introduction of first trimester antenatal diagnosis** of the fetus in 1982 and with the number of trained counsellors that became available. (*Ref 11*)

THALASSAEMIA

For beta thalassaemia there has been a high uptake since prenatal diagnosis first became established in 1977. By 1984 **the expected number of children affected with thalassaemia major had fallen by approximately 50%, as a result of antenatal screening with counselling.** There has been no further fall in the past five years: most newly diagnosed affected children are now of Pakistani or other South Asian origin, and there is evidence that in many cases antenatal screening and counselling in a language both parents can understand had not been provided (*Ref 12*).

Other important factors include the time of first booking which may be delayed either because of appointments being issued late or may be determined by patient preference and appears to differ between racial groups and socio-economic groups, see Appendix 4 (extracted from *Ref 13*),

Table 3. SCREENING FOR THE HAEMOGLOBINOPATHIES

Type of screening	What are the objectives of screening?	What sort of screening programme is recommended for:	
		Sickle cell disorder	Thalassaemia
Preconceptional	• to give women and their partners information about their genetic status, so that they can make informed choices about possible future pregnancies (SCD & thalassaemia)	selective	selective
Antenatal	• to give women and their partners information about their genetic status, so that they can make an informed choice about whether to have prenatal diagnosis (SCD & thalassaemia)	selective if antenatal population includes < 15% ethnic minorities at risk of SCD	universal mean cell haemoglobin (MCH)
	• identification of trait	universal if antenatal population includes > 15% ethnic minorities at risk of SCD	
Neonatal	• to identify all neonates with SCD, so that they can be enrolled into a programme of systematic follow-up and care	selective if antenatal population includes < 15% ethnic minorities at risk of SCD	Most thalassaemia major detected but not thalassaemia carriers
	• identification of trait	universal if antenatal population includes > 15% ethnic minorities at risk of SCD	

All individuals with a low MCH must be followed-up by the haematology laboratory to check for iron deficiency as well as thalassaemia trait. (Iron deficiency can lead to difficulty in assessment of thalassaemia trait and needs to be corrected before repeat tests for the trait.)

Figure 3. HOW ANTENATAL SCREENING SHOULD WORK

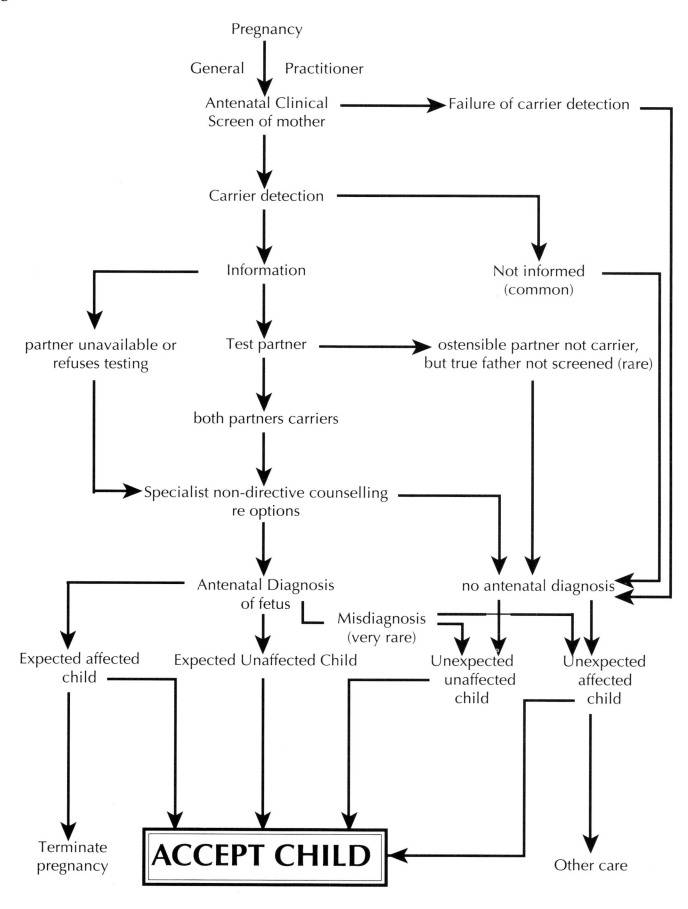

CONTINUED COUNSELLING

NEONATAL SCREENING

PURPOSE

The primary objective of neonatal screening is to identify children with SCD, in order to provide advice and protection, and particularly by starting prophylactic penicillin (Ref 14 and see section 8). It will also identify all sickle cell carrier babies which will require counselling and family studies. **This does not apply to alpha or beta thalassaemia. Babies who carry beta thalassaemia trait cannot be reliably identified by neonatal screening.** An organised neonatal screening programme is highly beneficial in increasing the awareness of health service staff and of the community at risk.

METHODS

Samples from the neonate can be examined either using a spot from the Guthrie card, usually performed at 6 days, or by using a capillary method. Both methods were considered by the Working Party. It was felt that there was little difference between the two in terms of value for money. **It is not advisable to use cord blood because of risk of contamination by maternal blood.**

Figure 3 shows that, with effective antenatal screening all pregnant carriers will be detected and informed. **However, owing to the difficulties of clearly identifying both parents genotype, all babies who have one or both parents from an ethnic group at risk of SCD should be tested.** It has been suggested (Ref 15) that **where the relevant ethnic group at risk is greater than 15% all neonates should be tested** because of the high level of interethnic marriage. The figure is based on research in one District and further research is necessary to establish whether a different figure is more appropriate. Table 4 shows the boroughs with more than 15% ethnic minority populations and Table 5 those with less than 15% but more than 5% ethnic minorities. It should be noted that sometimes babies are not followed-up when, for example, they are transferred to intensive care soon after birth. These concerns need to be addressed locally.

PROTOCOL

Each district requires a protocol to determine which neonates require screening. Midwives need to be made aware of this. In addition there may be difficulties where obstetric and paediatric services are provided by different units. These concerns may be addressed by the use of a designated co-ordinator. **It is essential that parents and GPs are informed of the results of the neonatal screening** and the implications of these results. It is therefore important for there to be good communication between health professionals caring for new mothers whether community or hospital based, for example, the antenatal clinic, community midwife, GP and community paediatrician. Districts and Regions have reported their experience of both universal and selective neonatal screening (*Ref 14, 15*).

ACCEPTABILITY

Screening must be acceptable to individuals with regard to the information it may provide, which may sometimes be alarming. It must also be **acceptable to communities**, and to their cultural and religious views, in view of the psychological stress and stigmatization which may occur (*Ref 13*). **Screening must be specific, sensitive and reliable.** Ideally it should also be cheap in relation to the benefits offered.

ETHICS

Ethical principles need to be observed. The individual must be allowed to choose whether or not to be screened. Choice must be informed by knowledge of the significance of screening for health benefit, including reproductive outcome, and also of any possible disadvantages of screening. **Confidentiality must always be preserved**. These considerations mean that education programmes directed at the population should be introduced before screening is begun. Pilot studies are needed to establish community attitudes and responses, and to determine the means of organisation. **Services available need to be monitored**. It would be useful to have national guidance on policy and standards for screening (*Ref 16*).

PSYCHOLOGICAL ASPECTS OF SCREENING

There has been relatively little recent work on psychological aspects of screening for SCD and thalassaemia in the UK, particularly when compared with the amount of research into antenatal screening for Down's syndrome and spina bifida. However some of the results from these other screening programmes are useful in planning screening for SCD and thalassaemia. The main themes that emerge from the studies to date are given below.

POPULATIONS AT RISK GIVEN INACCURATE/INAPPROPRIATE INFORMATION

As many as one third of women offered maternal serum alpha-fetoprotein screening for open-neural tube defects and Down's syndrome do not know whether they have undergone the test (Ref 17). Part of the reason for this limited understanding is the minimal and inaccurate information sometimes provided by health professionals (*Refs 18, 19*).

PRESSURE TO UNDERGO TESTS

Despite the recommendations of the 1989 Royal College of Physician's report on antenatal diagnosis and genetic screening (Ref 20) that decisions to undergo tests should be made by individuals on the basis of full information, **some women report feeling under pressure to undergo tests** (Ref 17). This feeling is substantiated by studies using tape-recordings of consultations in which routine antenatal tests are presented by obstetricians (*Ref 18*).

EFFECT OF TESTS ON INDIVIDUALS

Studies in screening for risk of cardiovascular disease suggest that **the impact of testing is influenced by how the test is presented**, and in particular about the information provided about the meaning of a positive result. Studies reporting the impact of carrier or antenatal testing need to be interpreted within the context of how the screening programme was organised.

Carrier testing for recessively inherited conditions such as SCD is associated with raised anxiety, and concerns about future health which for some are evident many years after carrier detection (Ref 21). Recent studies of carrier detection for cystic fibrosis during pregnancy suggests that these effects are short-lived if only one of the parents is found to be a carrier. Studies of parents who have an antenatal diagnosis and choose to have a termination when the child is affected show reactions of grief, mixed with relief.

We know little about the psychological effects on carriers who have children, having chosen not to undergo antenatal diagnosis; or for those who are diagnosed antenatally, but opt not to have a termination. There is a clear need for research.

Table 4: Boroughs within counties with more than 15% ethnic minority population

	Percentage of population that is non-white
Brent	44.8
Newham	42.3
Tower Hamlets	35.6
Hackney	33.6
Ealing	32.3
Birmingham	31.5
Lambeth	30.3
Haringey	29.0
Leicester	28.5
Slough	27.7
Harrow	26.2
Waltham Forest	25.6
Hounslow	24.4
Southwark	24.4
Lewisham	22.0
Westminster, City of	21.4
Redbridge	21.4
Wandsworth	20.0
Luton	19.8
Islington	18.9
Wolverhampton	18.6
Barnet	18.4
Croydon	17.6
Hammersmith & Fulham	17.5
Merton	16.3
Bradford	15.6
Kensington & Chelsea	15.6
Blackburn	15.4

Inner London Boroughs–Average 25.6
Outer London Boroughs–Average 19.7

* By late summer similar figures will be available by health authority.

Table 5: Boroughs with less than 15% but more than 5% ethnic minorities

	Percentage of population that is non-white
Sandwell	14.7
Enfield	14.1
Greenwich	12.7
Manchester	12.6
Hillingdon	12.3
Coventry	11.8
Nottingham	10.8
Kirklees	10.7
Pendle	10.3
Preston	10.2
North Bedfordshire	10.1
Watford	9.9
Derby	9.7
Walsall	9.6
Reading	9.5
Bolton	9.3
Oxford	9.2
Oldham	8.7
Kingston 'on Thames	8.6
Gravesham	8.4
Wycombe	8.3
Crawley	8.0
Rochdale	7.9
Peterborough	7.4
City of London	7.3
Wellingborough	7.2
Barking & Dagenham	6.8
Forest Heath	5.9
Charnwood	6.2
Northampton	5.9
Hyndburn	5.9
Sutton	5.9
Cambridge	5.9
Milton Keynes	5.8
Bexley	5.8
Gloucester	5.7
Epsom & Ewell	5.7
Warwick	5.6
Burnley	5.5
Richmond 'on Thames	5.5
North Hertfordshire	5.5
Trafford	5.4
Woking	5.4
Bristol	5.1

RECOMMENDATIONS

PRECONCEPTIONAL

- *Preconceptional carrier diagnosis should be encouraged and GPs have a significant part to play in this.*

ANTENATAL

- *If the population coming through the antenatal clinic is composed of 15% or more ethnic minorities at risk of SCD, there should be universal antenatal screening (ideally before 10 weeks into pregnancy) and neonatal screening . In other circumstances selective screening should be targeted appropriately.*

- *A co-ordinated antenatal screening programme, including the haemoglobinopathies, should be supported.*

NEONATAL

- *The Guthrie card and the capillary method are equally good methods for neonatal screening.*

- *Cord blood samples should be avoided for neonatal screening.*

OPPORTUNISTIC

- *All patients from ethnic minorities at risk of SCD should be screened pre-operatively unless written records show this has been done already.*

- *FHSAs should suggest GPs to include assessment of risk of haemoglobinopathy in new patients joining their practices.*

GENERAL

- *Individuals should be informed if they are being tested, their names recorded and they should be informed of the result in writing whether it is **positive or negative**.*

- *All GPs with significant numbers of the relevant ethnic groups on their lists should be encouraged to take part in haemoglobinopathy screening.*

- *If there is doubt whether the mother or the father of the child is at risk of haemoglobinopathy the individual should be screened.*

- *Research is needed to determine at what frequency of population at risk of haemoglobinopathy it is appropriate to do universal neonatal screening. Further consideration needs to be given to the notification of people who are confirmed to be negative.*

- *Research is needed particularly in the area of screening for SCD and thalassaemia to determine how decisions are made about testing, and the effects of being tested and declining testing.*

SECTION 4 • COUNSELLING

Many families affected by SCD and thalassaemia bitterly complain about the failure of health professionals to provide them with information both before their child was born and following the diagnosis. The working party was surprised to read the following in a text published as recently as 1976:

"Sickle-cell anaemia is not of great consequence to us in the context of genetic counselling in the United Kingdom. The sickling trait and sickle cell anaemia appear to be confined to peoples of African and Eastern origin."(Ref 22)

NEEDS OF FAMILIES

There is now increasing **recognition of the significance of counselling needs of families** affected by haemoglobinopathies. These needs are outlined below (*see Ref 23*):

- information in **appropriate languages and appropriate terms** before, during and after screening and diagnosis of the trait and the disorder.

- **health professionals** in the primary health care team and within hospitals who advise these families must have **detailed knowledge and skills**.

- support and information should respect the cultural backgrounds and ethhnic customs of the families.

- **non-directive genetic counselling and follow-up** and support regardless of the couple's decision, i.e. acceptance or refusal of antenatal diagnosis or possible termination of pregnancy.

- **monitoring of the quality** of in-patient and out-patient care as perceived by families and professionals.

A Confidential Enquiry into Counselling for Genetic Disorders is currently underway as part of the Royal College of Physician's clinical audit programme funded by the Department of Health. One of the disorders being studied is thalassaemia (Appendix 5).

HAEMOGLOBINOPATHY COUNSELLING

The last decade has seen the emergence of clinical nurse specialists involved in providing information and counselling about SCD and thalassaemia. The range of responsibilities that haemoglobinopathy counsellors may undertake, is set out in *Ref 24.*

The first such post was established in Brent in 1979. A survey of haemoglobinopathy counsellors has recently been undertaken (*Ref 25*). A summary table based on the report is given at Appendix 6.

Counselling and screening can also be undertaken as a health promotion activity within primary care. A major advantage is that having initially identified a couple at risk of haemoglobinopathy, a screening cascade, involving other family members, often develops. GPs are in the fortunate position of looking after whole families, which is less common in hospital practice. They are in a specially good position to integrate the other health needs of those with haemoglobinopathies. **Counsellors are required both as part of the multi-professional team of the hospital and in the community.**

RECOMMENDATIONS

- *All Staff involved with haemoglobinopathies should be trained in giving accurate information. Providers should ensure that health professionals, midwives, for example, are adequately trained before undertaking non-directive counselling.*

- *Designated counsellors should be properly trained and the counselling service must be co-ordinated with other aspects of the management of the haemoglobinopathies. In areas with small numbers of people at risk this work may be combined with other responsibilities.*

- *Counsellors should speak appropriate languages, wherever possible.*

- *Counsellors should assist self help groups to provide help for affected families in the community.*

- *Haemoglobinopathy counsellors should be available in sufficient numbers to ensure that the needs of both primary health care and hospitals are met.*

- *Research is needed into the most effective and appropriate methods of delivering haemoglobinopathy counselling services.*

SECTION 5 • SICKLE CELL DISORDER

PRIMARY CARE

BACKGROUND

The diagnosis, management and aftercare of patients with SCD and thalassaemia had long been considered by general practitioners to be the province of specialist secondary care services. More recently, interested general practitioners have begun to explore the contribution general practitioners might make to the care of those with these disorders.

The majority of general practitioners, even those working in urban areas, are unlikely to identify a single patient with overt haemoglobinopathy. This situation is changing with the increased migration of groups at risk. **It is likely that by the end of the millennium most GPs in urban areas will have contact with one or more families affected by the trait or disorder.** With increasing intermarriage, haemoglobinopathy genes will become more widely distributed among all ethnic groups.

SICKLE CELL TRAIT

The carrier state for SCD is sickle cell trait. While this is a benign condition, not affecting life expectancy, it needs to be identified as it has implications for management of general anaesthesia and some surgical procedures, such as tourniquets. Therefore it is important that sickle cell trait is recognised so that patients and those responsible for their clinical management are aware and firm reassurance can be given in respect of the clinical prognosis. This is in addition to benefits for genetic counselling referred to earlier.

NUMBERS OF PATIENTS

Currently a typical general practitioner working in an inner city area might expect to have 1900 patients registered on the NHS list. If 20% of these were of Afro-Caribbean origin and another 20% of Asian and Middle Eastern origin then we might expect that GP to care for one patient with a SCD and one with beta-thalassaemia requiring active treatment. The number of carriers is likely to be unknown but can be estimated at around 50 for sickle cell trait and 20 for beta thalassaemia trait. However at current incidence rates this general practitioner is likely to register a new patient with a SCD every five years and one leaves the practice or dies every ten years. This needs to be compared with the incidence of disorders such as coronary artery disease (4 new patients per year and 15 current patients requiring continued care), cancer of the breast (3 new patients per year, 10 current), depression (8 new patients, 20 current).

Anecdotal evidence suggests there is at least one practice in most major cities in the UK which is "taking an interest" in patients with the haemoglobinopathies. Although a "body of expertise" appears to be developing among a small group of interested GPs, the majority of GPs even in areas of high prevalence will expect a specialised secondary care service to manage all aspects of patient care related to the haemoglobinopathy. **Models of care** for patients with haemoglobinopathies will differ depending on whether they are registered either with a practitioner with **minimal** involvement or a practice with **maximum** interest in managing such patients.

PATIENT EXPECTATIONS

Patients will expect the GP to have a basic knowledge of SCD and its complications. They will also expect an understanding of the distress that previous experiences of the disorder might have created and for the GP to be sympathetic and supportive when further anxieties are expressed. The patients might also reasonably expect the practitioner to be aware of guidelines or policies for managing patients with acute illness or complications, e.g. sickle cell crises, aplastic crises and major infections, and to be able to provide immediate analgesia and urgent referrals. He or she should be familiar with the referral procedure for the specialist secondary care unit the patient generally uses. This is particularly important in the case of newly diagnosed infants with SCD where referral to a specialist clinic is necessary, and **prophylactic penicillin needs to be prescribed and compliance monitored.** The practitioner should also be aware of, and if requested participate in, follow up and management of chronic aspects of the disorders. This might include the provision of family planning, immunisation and other health promotion procedures including counselling and screening. The practitioner might also consider managing routine prescribing for these disorders. However written and oral evidence to the working party stated that many patients were dissatisfied with GPs' knowledge of their condition and preferred to bypass them and deal directly with the hospital.

In determining policies in respect of care by GPs for haemoglobinopathy patients the following elements need to be incorporated. All GPs treating haemoglobinopathy patients need to take into account:

(a) Policies should be **patient centred** and heed the needs of the patient's family.

(b) **Co-operation and co-ordination with specialist centres and counselling services**, where they exist, should be clearly expressed and implemented. If these services are close by, shared care needs to be considered.

(c) Practice policies will need to be flexible and audited to **assure patients of continuity of care and sensitivity to their special needs**.

AMBULANCE SERVICE

Many sickle cell **patients develop a good rapport with a particular hospital**. They prefer to be admitted to that hospital, even though **it may not be nearest to them**. Provided this will not unreasonably prolong the ambulance's journey, **many ambulance services are prepared to take a patient to the preferred hospital** (*Ref 26*). Purchasers need to consider these preferences in placing contracts. In some cases there have been difficulties which have led patients to book their own taxis in order to ensure admission to their chosen hospital. If analgesia prescribed by the GP or self-administered is insufficient, **ambulance crews may provide Entonox** on the journey to the A&E department.

PROTOCOLS FOR MANAGEMENT IN HOSPITAL

ACCIDENT AND EMERGENCY (A&E)

When the patient is on route to hospital urgent contact with the haematologist may be necessary. Initial assessment in the A&E department will determine the gravity of the presenting episode. Urgent contact should be made with the haematologist to plan further management. A local protocol is necessary.

At present A&E departments have different guidelines for managing patients in sickle cell crisis. It is recommended that **all guidelines should follow the basic aims of fast, adequate relief of pain with strong analgesics, a reduction of precipitating factors by rehydration, warmth and additional oxygen as necessary and the establishment of the aetiology of the pain.** To facilitate the introduction of such guidelines the British Association For Accident and Emergency Medicine is preparing model guidelines based on the principles contained in this document to serve as a basis for local policy.

If patients are known or are carrying a **haemoglobinopathy card** they should be **treated immediately with the drug shown on the card** if it is apparent to the receiving clinician that they are having a crisis or starting one. If patients are not known, or not carrying a card, they should be given Entonox and possibly a **single dose** of a strong analgesic such as an opiate or non-steroidal anti-inflammatory drugs (NSAIDs) if indicated and allowed by local guidelines until the diagnosis of sickle cell crisis is made, when continuous analgesics (usually opiates) will be required until pain control is established. Training and education of staff are required to enable them to manage the anxious patient by reassurance, and to give adequate pain relief for the severity of pain with which they present, rather than treat anxiety with anxiolytics.

INPATIENT HOSPITAL CARE

The specific components of care provided by a hospital for SCD will depend on various factors. The **major criteria** will be the **number of patients with SCD served** and the consequent expertise and facilities available. Several local guides to management have been produced (*Ref 27, 28*).

In hospital units with a large number of haemoglobinopathy patients, it may be helpful to have data on individual patients stored on a computer. Access to this information should be restricted to clinicians looking after patients in the unit and to the A&E Department.

Important aspects to be included in local protocols are detailed below. All the facilities should be available in a specialist haemoglobinopathy unit but items C2 and C3 are not essential for ordinary hospitals which may need to admit patients with SCD as an emergency.

A. OVERALL REQUIREMENTS

1. Each provider to have a **scheme of management** for SCD under the direction of an **identified clinician**, usually a haematologist with a nominated deputy. **The number of patients with the disorder regularly seen at neighbouring provider units may indicate a need for a haemoglobinopathy centre – see Section 12 and Table 7 .**

2. Outpatient care either by the unit or with satisfactory referral to another unit

3. Inpatient care

4. Laboratory support (24 hours availability)

5. Antenatal/maternity supervision

6. Paediatric facilities

7. Social and psychological support (see Appendix 8)

8. Evaluation and audit (see Section 11)

B. BASIC REQUIREMENTS OF (CONTINUING) OUTPATIENT CARE

1. Each provider to have a **scheme of management** for the haemoglobinopathies under the direction of an **identified clinician**, with a nominated deputy.

2. Facilities for children and adults

3. Planned regular clinical review

4. Provision of haemoglobinopathy cards

5. Good communication and integration with primary health care

6. Supervision of prophylaxis, antibiotics etc.

7. Initiation and supervision of therapy

   a. Transfusion regime

   b. Iron chelation therapy

8. Social and psychological support

9. Fertility/contraception advice

10. Identification of, and provision of, arrangements for management of complications, e.g. renal, ophthalmic, delayed puberty, orthopaedic.

C. BASIC REQUIREMENTS OF INPATIENT CARE

1. Rapid direct access to assessment and treatment, i.e. 'Hospital Admissions Policy'

2. Designated unit with designated trained nurses and doctors   }   see * above

3. Pulse oximeter on the designated unit   }   see * above

4. 24 hour laboratory support

5. Written guidelines available on the general management of clinical situations including rehydration and pain relief
   (see Section 6)

   a. painful crises (usually musculo-skeletal)

   b. chest syndrome

   c. aplastic crises

   d. stroke and other CNS manifestations

   e. sequestration crises

   f. infections

      i. pulmonary

      ii. bone

      iii. septicaemia

6. Surgical and both general and local anaesthetic policies. (*Ref 29*)

D. BASIC LABORATORY PROVISION REQUIRED WITH APPROPRIATE QUALITY CONTROL

1. Haematology

Full blood count   }THROUGHOUT 24 HOURS
Sickle screen (solubility test)   }
Blood transfusion   }
Reticulocyte count
Hb electrophoresis – within 24 hours
Serum ferritin

2. Medical microbiology

Culture of urine, throat and stool specimens
CSF analysis
Blood culture

3. Chemical pathology

Blood gases	} THROUGHOUT 24 HOURS
Urea and electrolytes	}

4. X-ray

Chest X-ray	} THROUGHOUT 24 HOURS
Straight Abdomen	}

E. BASIC REQUIREMENTS OF ANTENATAL/MATERNITY CARE

1. Designated consultant obstetricians to collaborate with designated clinician

2. Agreed management policies during pregnancy and post-partum, e.g. pain relief and transfusion

3. Regular fetal assessment – growth retardation

4. Anaesthetic collaboration

F. SERVICE NEEDS OF CHILDREN WITH SICKLE CELL DISORDER (see Section 8)

G. OTHER CONSIDERATIONS

Management of specific problems in SCD within the UK has been considered in several publications (Ref 28-36). These give sufficient detail to alert the non-specialist to clinical situations which may be encountered and which on occasion may be life-threatening if not correctly managed. In case of difficulty it is advisable to ask for advice from haematologists working in specialist units.

Disabilities as a result of complications of SCD such as stroke, require multidisciplinary assessment. **Access is required to rehabilitation therapy** and provision may be needed for special educational needs and advice given about appropriate social security payments.

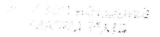

RECOMMENDATIONS

- *Purchasing Authorities with a high proportion of ethnic minorities at risk of haemoglobinopathies should consider commissioning comprehensive centres from provider units.*

- *In comprehensive centres there should be designated beds and clinical nurse specialists, and counsellors should be part of the team looking after the patient in hospital.*

- *Guidelines for the management of acute sickle cell crisis should be available and prominently displayed in every A&E department. These guidelines should have been prepared in co-operation with relevant departments, e.g., haematology, paediatric and A&E itself and should cover the rapid relief of acute pain and the management of precipitating factors and life-threatening complications.*

- *There should be good communication between the hospital consultants and the GPs in the area to provide continuity of care. There is merit in FHSAs recognising GPs and their practices who are prepared to take special interest in the primary care management of those patients with haemoglobinopathies in co-operation with specialist services.*

- *An identified clinician, with a nominated deputy, should have responsibility for overall patient care.*

- *Wherever possible patients' wishes should be taken into account when deciding where their treatment should take place.*

- *The patient and the hospital consultant should mutually agree which analgesic the patient may require for an acute crisis. Adequate information should be available to the patient with regard to drug potency, side effects and problems of accumulation and metabolites. The name of this drug and its dose and route of administration should be given on the haemoglobinopathy card and on the patient's records.*

- *If patients are known or carrying a haemoglobinopathy card they should be treated immediately with the drug shown on the card if it is apparent to the receiving physician that they are having a crisis or starting one. If patients are not known or not carrying a card they should be given Entonox or a single dose of a strong analgesic until further information indicates that they are having a sickle cell crisis. Patients must be made to feel comfortable on arrival in A&E departments in order to reduce the need for anxiolytics.*

EFFECT ON INDIVIDUALS

Patient perception of pain and its control have been considered by various authors. Some of these articles are in the scientific literature (*Ref 37, 38*) but perhaps even more important are documents produced by patients (*Ref 39*). The latter gives an overall picture of the acute and chronic pain problems and also consider other, non-pharmacological alternatives, which may be of great help to an individual. These include a reassuring comfortable environment in which to be treated with staff trained to assess pain and maintain pain relief. They also give graphic, distressing descriptions of the impressions of pain in sickle cell crisis.

"The problem with Casualty is that you arrive in an awful lot of pain, then they call a doctor; (I always tend to call the haematology doctor so that they are standing by when I get there). Then in Casualty – this is no disrespect to Casualty staff – they have to put up a drip first and then they want to ask your history details, which is already on your file and which they already know. It is very difficult to keep still while the doctor puts in a drip and you are in so much pain. To me the most important thing is getting the pain under control and then you can relax and have the drip put in, you can answer questions and you can be examined. But when they want to examine you first, put the drip in and ask all these questions, it is very very difficult. You sometimes tend to lash out at them and they think you are being awkward." Sharon Edwards (*Ref 1*)

This quotation highlights the problem from the patient's perspective and the dilemmas faced by A&E staff without adequate documentation.

SEVERITY OF PAIN

Severe pain is the main complicating feature of sickle crisis. Since this is a subjective symptom and often few clinical signs are evident, this may lead to **difficulties in diagnosis** unless the clinician is aware of the possible cause. This is **particularly relevant in those districts where few sickle cell patients are seen routinely**. Patients may feel that their GP or doctors in A&E departments do not appreciate the severity of the pain, and the need for opiate analgesia in some circumstances. The frequency of painful crises with consequent time off work may lead to unemployment and unfairly labelling patients as lazy or worse (*Ref 37*).

CONTROLLED DRUGS

A&E medical staff have large numbers of patients requiring **immediate attention** and with a variety of demands. **Decisions may be difficult** and need to be made speedily and medical practitioners need to be circumspect about **prescribing controlled drugs**. However, there is evidence that a **strict protocol** can enable those patients that really need such drugs to be **treated effectively**.

IDENTIFICATION OF PROBLEMS

The pain of a sickle cell crisis cannot be treated adequately unless certain problems are identified:

a)   the diagnosis of SCD is made

b)   the severity of the pain is assessed

c)   the age and weight of the patient is sought to determine drug dosage and suitable route of administration

d)   previous analgesia, its type and dosage, is ascertained and problems of toxicity and potential addiction are considered

e)   other system disorder and drugs, for example: renal failure and drug excretion; enzyme inducing drugs (such as alcohol and anti epileptic drugs) which may increase metabolite formation with opioid drugs and precipitate convulsions.

OBJECTIVES OF PAIN MANAGEMENT

The **objectives of pain management** for sickle cell crisis relate to **three stages**:

1.   Acutely (in A&E)

2.   In patient admission

3.   Long-term management and
     all should be subject to audit processes.

PAIN MANAGEMENT IN A&E

When the patient is starting a sickle cell crisis and is in acute, severe, pain, **relief of this pain must be fast and adequate**. If there is dehydration, e.g. after excessive exercise has precipitated the crisis and where there is some degree of peripheral circulatory failure, intramuscular drugs may not be well absorbed and it may be difficult to establish intravenous access. Intravenous access is probably the best route to allow rapid titration of an opioid to reduce pain to an acceptable level and to hydrate the patient. Children may require alternative routes. If pain relief is inadequate or side effects such as nausea limit the dose of analgesic which can be given, secondary analgesics such as NSAIDs may be indicated. Although NSAIDs produce renal prostaglandin inhibition it is very unlikely that a single dose will cause a problem (Ref 40–42). Partial agonist and antagonist opioid drugs, e.g. buprenorphine, pentazocine are not recommended for treatment of acute pain before transfer to hospital, e.g. by the GP. Drug interactions should be considered (see section (e) above).

Sickle cell crisis may have been precipitated by dehydration, cold or hypoxia. These should be reversed in the acute situation by nursing the patient in a warm environment and administering fluids. In those patients with hypoxia, for example, chest syndrome or severe anaemia, oxygen by mask is indicated initially. Entonox (a 50:50 mixture of nitrous oxide and oxygen) can be used to provide both pain relief and additional oxygenation.

The cause of the pain and differential diagnosis should be made in this acute situation and **patient examination may be helped by administering analgesia first**.

INPATIENT MANAGEMENT OF PAIN

There are three objectives on in-patient admission. These are:

(i)   maintenance of analgesia

(ii)   monitoring of pain and response to analgesia

(iii)   removal of precipitating factors of a crisis

The pain protocol available for stage (i) should also reflect management in stage (ii) where a specific acute pain team may be asked for advice or may treat a patient. The chosen regime should therefore be acceptable to all departments involved in the patient's management. Pain assessments can be made by trained staff and a variety of methods chosen depending on the availability of staff and equipment (*Ref 43*).

LONG-TERM MANAGEMENT OF PAIN

Long term management of pain relief will require an individualised pain plan for acute admissions. Where, for example, joint complications are associated with chronic pain, multidisciplinary care should be given with adequate patient understanding. **Information on the prevention of painful episodes and self medication should be part of the counselling process.**

DRUGS USED IN SICKLE CELL CRISES

Various drugs have been used to try to alleviate pain in sickle cell crisis. Anxieties have been raised about excessive dosage, especially when opioids are given by different medical practitioners along the route from home to hospital and the formation of toxic metabolites of pethidine and morphine-like drugs (*Ref 44, 45*). There are no randomised clinical trials of opioid analgesic use in sickle cell crisis reported in the scientific literature. Historically, **pethidine has been the opiate of choice**. Although **its metabolite nor-pethidine is a stimulant and has the potential of inducing convulsions the degree of risk has not been defined. Because of its efficacy patients and medical practitioners are often unwilling to change to other drugs.** Patients may also complain of the sedative or emetic effects of morphine. The present situation may change with the introduction of more specific analgesics without these unwanted effects. As a working recommendation, **patients** with the advice of their medical practitioners should be able to **make an informed choice depending on their response to the available drugs** and **new patients, such as children, should probably avoid pethidine in an acute sickle cell crisis.**

RECOMMENDATIONS

- *Each patient should have an individual plan for the management of pain. Individuals should be given enough information to make informed decisions about their choice of drug.*

- *Pain relief should be fast and adequate and monitored by trained staff. A pain management protocol is necessary in hospitals which treat patients in sickle cell crisis and is essential in specialist haemoglobinopathy units.*

- *In acute crisis, patients may be given short acting oral morphine by GPs because it is reversible.*

- *The GP has a role in the management of chronic pain, for example, for patients with avascular hip necrosis, and also in the provision of self-administered analgesia for early crisis management*

- *Partial agonist and antagonist opioid drugs e.g. buprenorphine, pentazocine, are not recommended for treatment of acute pain before to transfer to hospital, e.g., by the GP.*

- *Entonox is a useful analgesic for use in ambulances and A&E. It should not be used at home.*

- *Randomised clinical trials are needed to test the relative value of pethidine and morphine and new drugs.*

BACKGROUND

" It's very frustrating when I arrange to have time off for my transfusion only to arrive at the ward and be told that although the blood is ready, there is no bed available. On one occasion my sister and I had to go in on the same day, the nurse phoned me to say that there was only one bed available and only one of us could go. At times like this I feel vulnerable and like an orphan beggar with nowhere to go and having to beg for a bed in order to be treated." (*Ref 46*)

"...I am sixteen and just finished my fifth form studies... I hope to go onto College and do a Graphic Design course. I am the eldest of two children, I have a sister... who is fourteen. No, she doesn't have Thalassaemia in case any of you reading this are wondering.

"I have always been very active, taken part in sports at school and out of school, I enjoy playing football, tennis and snooker, and I can honestly say having Thalassaemia has not hindered my life in any way. Of course I don't particularly like going to hospital for my treatment and I look forward to the day when we can throw our "pumps" away and take tablets to get rid of the iron, but other than that I consider my life is pretty normal." (*Ref 46*)

These two quotations give an indication of the marked differences in patients' perceptions of thalassaemia. Perceptions will depend, in part, on patients' experiences of management of their condition. There may be major dissatisfaction with health care and this may dominate a person's life or it may be a relatively small irritant with which one has to put up but which does not significantly affect a person's behaviour and aspirations.

Although many of the factors mentioned below are the same as those covered for SCD, the working party considered it useful to have a **separate list of requirements for thalassaemia major**.

This report has referred earlier to aspects of screening and counselling for thalassaemia major and for thalassaemia trait.

Most of the **clinical work** in respect of thalassaemia major is **hospital-based** but primary care has a part to play in the support and encouragement of the patient and the patient's family. It is uncommon for thalassaemia major patients to need emergency admission in respect of their haemoglobinopathy.

In general, thalassaemia is a condition with predictable needs whereas patients with SCD often have acute episodes which cannot be foreseen.

The main cause of emergency admission in thalassaemia is a pyrexia of undetermined origin, a "PUO". This must be taken very seriously as it may indicate a potentially overwhelming infection. This is a risk both in splenectomised patients, and in any patient on regular desferrioxamine. Such patients are particularly susceptible to *Yersinia enterocolitica* septicaemia.

Appendix 7 is an example of recommendations for treatment of thalassaemia major to ensure good health and quality of life, in the long as well as the short term.

TRANSFUSION AND CHELATION

Regular (approximately monthly) blood transfusions are required. However, regular transfusion leads to transfusional iron overload, which if untreated may cause death in the mid teens. It can be controlled by the iron chelating drug desferrioxamine. This is usually infused subcutaneously over 8 – 10 hours/night on 5 nights a week, from a portable syringe driver ("the pump").

OTHER CONSIDERATIONS

Splenectomy may be necessary. Endocrine complications and disturbances of pubertal growth and sexual development may need specific treatment.

Treatment is highly predictable and patients need continuity of clinical care and psychosocial support. Appendix 8 gives details of the sort of psychosocial support needed. Evidence suggests that patient compliance with treatment can prove difficult particularly during the teenage years when patients do not wish to be different from their peers and complain about the "unfairness" of their situation. Unfortunately this can lead to increased morbidity and even mortality.

IMPACT OF TREATMENT

Treatment needs to be organised to minimise disturbance of patients' daily lives. Transfusions ideally should be arranged for a time that suits the family, including evenings or weekends. Evening outpatient visits and transfusions would be welcome to avoid interrupting education and work. However it is recognised that in many instances these ideals cannot be achieved. There are fewer staff available in the evenings and at weekends. House staff may be caring for a very large number of patients and may not know the haemoglobinopathy patients. In some wards blood transfusions are not allowed in the late evenings or at night because the patients cannot be adequately monitored. Delays in setting up transfusions were a common complaint and thought needs to be given to reduce these as much as possible and explanations need to be given if these are unavoidable.

CONTINUITY OF CARE

Continuity of patient care by the same physician and nursing staff in the same outpatient and inpatient facilities is desirable. Patients should be seen at regular intervals and registrars who see the patient at other times should be fully aware of the individual plan of treatment for that patient.
Details of the routine care are given below:

A. OVERALL REQUIREMENTS

1. Where relevant: identification of haemoglobinopathy centres (depending on incidence of disease). Each centre should be under direction of an identified clinician and nominated deputy, usually a haematologist, responsible for the provision of:

2. Outpatient Care.

3. Inpatient Care – the use of specially trained nurses can help to facilitate continuity of care.

4. Laboratory support (24-hour availability).

5. Paediatric facilities.

6. Social and Psychological support.

7. Evaluation and audit (see Section 11)

B. BASIC REQUIREMENT OF (CONTINUING) OUTPATIENT CARE

1. Identified clinician responsible.

2. Facilities for children and adults.

3. Planned regular clinical review.

4. Provision of haemoglobinopathy cards.

5. Supervision of therapy

    a. Transfusion regime

    b. Iron Chelation therapy – provision of chelators and infusion pumps.

    c. Monitoring of growth and sexual development and function.

6. Good communication with primary health care.

7. Identification of complications

    a. Hepatic

    b. Cardiac

    c. Endocrine

    d. Fertility/Contraception advice.

8. Social and Psychological support.

C. BASIC REQUIREMENTS OF INPATIENT CARE

1. Designated Unit with designated nurses and doctors (where specialist centre exists)

2. 24-hour laboratory support.

3. Written guidelines available on general management of clinical situation.

D. BASIC LABORATORY PROVISION REQUIRED WITH APPROPRIATE QUALITY CONTROL

1. Haematology

    Full blood count   } THROUGHOUT 24 HOURS

    Blood transfusion   }

    Hb electrophoresis

    Serum ferritin

2. Medical Microbiology

    Culture of urine, throat and stool specimens

    Blood culture.

E. SERVICE NEEDS OF CHILDREN WITH THALASSAEMIA

    (see Section 8)

RECOMMENDATIONS

- *Mechanisms need to be developed to improve communication between the hospital consultants dealing with haemoglobinopathy and the primary health care team to provide continuity of care.*

- *An identified clinician, with a nominated deputy, should have responsibility for overall patient care.*

- *Wherever possible patients' wishes should be taken into account when deciding where their treatment should take place.*

- *There should be continuity of care in the hospital and the community.*

- *In specialist centres, there should be designated beds and clinical nurse specialists, and counsellors should be part of the team looking after the patient in hospital.*

- *Treatment needs to be organised to minimise disturbance of patients' daily lives as much as possible.*

- *Forward planning of patients' admissions should ensure that delays in setting up transfusions are avoided if at all possible. Patients should be provided with explanations for delay if it occurs.*

SECTION 8 • SPECIAL CONSIDERATIONS FOR THE CARE OF CHILDREN WITH HAEMOGLOBINOPATHIES

Sections 5 and 6 refer to general principles of management of SCD and associated pain, and Section 7 outlines principles of management of thalassaemia. However, management of children with haemoglobinopathies differs in some aspects from that of adults (*Ref 47, 48*). Earlier reference to this has been made in Section 5. In 1991 the Department of Health issued guidance (*Ref 47*) on the welfare of children and young people in hospital. This guidance is, of course, relevant when considering the care of children with haemoglobinopathies.

DIAGNOSIS

The importance of neonatal diagnosis of SCD has previously been stressed. Newborn babies with SCD have normal blood counts because of normal fetal haemoglobin production and **SCD often does not present clinically until after the first 3 months of life**, when fetal haemoglobin levels have declined towards adult concentrations. **The high early mortality from complications which are potentially preventable or treatable by, for example, use of prophylactic penicillin makes it essential to diagnose patients early**. The diagnosis needs to be made with great care and in particular the subtype of SCD can often not be clearly determined at birth. Differentiation of haemoglobin SS disease from S-beta-thalassaemia and sickle trait interacting with hereditary persistence of high fetal haemoglobin (SHPFH) can be very difficult, needing parental studies. It is very important that this difficulty is appreciated because misdiagnosis can – and indeed has – raised doubts about paternity which can have a devastating effect on the family. The diagnosis should always be confirmed by a second testing at 6 months.

SPECIFIC PROBLEMS

SICKLE CELL DISORDER

A high proportion of people with SCD are children and adolescents. Specific problems that need to be addressed in the case of children with SCD include **infection, enuresis, crises, growth and development, stroke and splenic sequestration**. The management of these complications require specialist knowledge and skill. These are best achieved by co-operation between interested haematologists and paediatricians although additional specialists should be involved at an early stage where their input would be useful, for example, the early involvement of an orthopaedic surgeon in the management of avascular hips. **Many children's wards provide open access to patients with SCD and their parents**. The management of pain in sickle cell crises needs to be adapted to children's needs (Appendix 9) and (*Ref 49*).

The major clinical management problems of this age group are:

Infections

Infections from *pneumococcus* and to a lesser extent *haemophilus influenzae* and *salmonella* occur from at least 3 months of age and measures are needed to encourage **compliance with penicillin prophylaxis**.   This is one of very few treatments strongly supported by research evidence and is often not undertaken despite the national reduction in morbidity and mortality which has followed introduction of this treatment.

However, compliance problems are major even in well run clinics and centres. **Pneumococcal vaccination is required**. Vaccination against Haemophilus B has now been introduced universally. GPs should ensure that child health surveillance (CHS) and immunisation is available to these children as to any others.

Acute painful crises

Acute painful crises require attention with age appropriate care (pulse oximetry with high dosage analgesia) and drug selection and dosage (see Section 6). As in adults, pain relief needs are often underestimated. Factors which may trigger crises and are avoidable include: exposure to cold and damp environment (including bedding resulting from the common complication of nocturnal enuresis); developed treatment, including fluids, of febrile illnesses; recognition of sleep hypoxia from upper airway obstruction (*Ref 50*); and avoidance of overstressing exercise at school. Preventive measures involve local authority housing, social service and education services as well as facilitating awareness amongst anaesthetic, dental and surgical specialties treating children.

Aplastic crises

This complication of SCD can occur at any age although it predominantly occurs in children and is associated with parvovirus infection. Following a 'flu-like' illness the marrow stops making red cells and this leads to a rapid deterioration of the anaemia which may be life-threatening. **Immediate intervention is indicated with blood transfusion**. If more than one child within a family has SCD, aplastic crises may occur in other children at the same time because of spread of infection.

Splenic and other sequestration syndromes

These syndromes present as an acute collapse with pain due to swelling of the spleen and may occur in early infancy. They require urgent referral to hospital and often need blood transfusion. These conditions may recur and so it is necessary to teach the parents how to recognise the symptoms at an early stage.

Stroke and other neurological impairment

The majority of strokes occur in childhood at a median age of 7 years and affect about 7 – 10% of children with a **high recurrence risk** (two-thirds within 3 years). **Early warning signs of stroke** (paraesthesia) **should be recognised by all involved**, including school nurses. Children with SCD and stroke should be immediately exchange transfused to minimise the risk of permanent damage and recurrence. Sub-clinical events without stroke (*Ref 51*) and after stroke (*Ref 52, 53*) may lead to more subtle neurological disability in the form of clumsiness or learning difficulties and leads to poor school performance compounded by frequent absences because of sickness; and decreased employment prospects.

Poor growth and delayed puberty

Poor growth and delayed puberty may lead to adolescent self esteem problems aggravated by such concerns at that age as enuresis, priapism, awareness of the implications of a genetic disorder, worries about sexual function or death; socialisation problems because of school loss, frequent illness, alcohol-provoked symptoms.

THALASSAEMIA

Many of the considerations are similar to those for SCD. However, the condition in the individual patient is more predictable and so management can be more precisely organised.

Transfusion and Chelation

Up to 5% of children with homozygous beta thalassaemia have a milder form of the disorder and may not need regular blood transfusion (thalassaemia intermedia). The remainder will be transfusion-dependent and have thalassaemia major. The decision to start regular transfusions is an important one that should not be taken too hastily, and requires careful assessment of the patient's clinical progress. Precise DNA genotyping is extremely helpful in differential diagnosis of thalassaemia major and intermedia, and should be carried out at an early stage. This will also be helpful should antenatal diagnosis be requested in subsequent pregnancies.

Children with thalassaemia major require regular blood transfusion. In addition, **chelation needs to be started by the age of 3 years.** Some patients with SCD also have frequent transfusions and need chelation. This requires co-operation between health professionals and the patient's family. Every endeavour should be made in arrangements for transfusion to **minimise disruption to school attendance and social life.** Children need much encouragement to persevere with chelation particularly during their early teens to avoid long-term harm due to iron deposition. Patients who have HLA matched siblings need to be considered for bone transplantation at an early age before tissue damage has occurred (*Ref 54, 55*).

SERVICE NEEDS OF CHILDREN WITH HAEMOGLOBINOPATHIES – ADDITIONAL TO THOSE OF ADULTS GIVEN IN SECTIONS 5,6 AND 7

A. DIAGNOSIS

1. Diagnosis **within the first 3 months offers optimal opportunities** for clinical management, counselling and health and social service support.

B. MULTIPROFESSIONAL MANAGEMENT

1. Clinics should have involvement of Consultant Paediatricians, including Consultant Paediatricians with special interest in Community Child Health and GPs, to ensure appropriate community (social service and education) linkages.

C. INFORMATION

1. Parents and carers

   Appropriate information, education and communication for parents and carers (including nursery teachers) is very important.

2. Health professionals

   GPs, health visitors, school nurses, consultant paediatricians and consultant paediatricians with special interest in Community Child Health also need appropriate information.

3. Social Services

   Social services will need medical advice from consultant paediatricians with special interest in Community Child Health and medical and nursing input to day care facilities including private child minders.

4. Education services

   Education services and teaching staff need support and information, for example, about the avoidance of excessive exercise in a cold environment in order to prevent the onset of a sickle cell crisis.

5. Housing Departments

   Environmental requirements need attention in home and school; for example, housing which is cold and damp can trigger a sickle cell crisis.

D ADOLESCENT TRANSFER

At adolescence transfer of care to an experienced adult physician, usually a haematologist, **should be planned jointly. This is to ensure continuity of treatment and to allow discussion and general agreement between physicians on particular aspects of management.**

RECOMMENDATIONS

- *Children with SCD should be given prophylactic penicillin from not later than 3 months old in addition to vaccination against pneumoccocus.*

- *Patients should be managed jointly by paediatricians and haematologists and the transfer at adolescence should be jointly planned.*

- *Where possible there should be a facility for direct admission to a designated children's ward.*

- *Facilities should be available for parents to stay overnight with their children.*

- *All children should be registered with a haemoglobinopathy centre*

- *All those linked with the care of children with haemoglobinopathies (including parents, teachers and health professionals) need to be made aware of these conditions and the requirements of children who have them*

SECTION 9 • EDUCATION

The multi-ethnic structure of society has brought about a need for knowledge of diseases and patterns of illness which differ from those commonly seen in the past. The haemoglobinopathies are a prime example of this. Knowledge of these conditions is particularly important in those areas where populations at risk comprise a significant proportion of the total population. **Different sections of society require varying amounts of information** and these are considered below.

GENERAL PUBLIC

The general public need to be aware of the existence of haemoglobinopathies as part of their general knowledge of health. In some geographical areas this may be particularly relevant as indicated previously. **Haemoglobinopathies may be featured in teaching on genetics in biology classes.** This must be done sensitively – e.g. by also considering other common genetic disorders such as cystic fibrosis – so that ethnic minorities do not become stigmatised. The approach in classes where some of the pupils are carriers or have major disorders needs even more careful consideration. Teachers in such situations need to be able to obtain guidance from health professionals on the best way to approach these potential difficulties.

COMMUNITIES AT RISK

Members of ethnic minorities at risk of haemoglobinopathies need much more information than other members of the general public. This needs to be in **appropriate terms and appropriate language**. Various publications have been issued by patient groups, local authorities and health authorities in the UK. These range from informed locally-produced documents, often photocopied, (*Ref 56 – 58*) to professional printed publications (*Ref 59 – 61*). Some publications are in the relevant mother tongue (*Ref 62*). There are also available publications produced in other countries e.g. USA (*Ref 63*) but which need to be read in context, in view of different provisions of health care.

HEALTH PROFESSIONALS

UNDERGRADUATE EDUCATION

Undergraduate education about haemoglobinopathies in medical schools is **variable**. The working party felt that where undergraduate teaching on haemoglobinopathies was currently adequate it was unnecessary to add any further teaching to the undergraduate curriculum though some change in organisation and emphasis might be beneficial. Undergraduates are taught about the haemoglobinopathies in a variety of courses, for example, genetics, haematology, general medicine. The overall content of the haemoglobinopathies taught in any given medical school often depends on the proportion of ethnic minorities in the population served. Members agreed that all undergraduates should have **educational objectives for the haemoglobinopathies**. This gives syllabus co-ordinators flexibility to tie the objectives into relevant courses as appropriate locally. Undergraduates would need to know about **diagnosis of patients and carriers, awareness of the groups at risk, how the disorders are inherited, options for diagnosis and subsequent action, and what treatment patients with haemoglobinopathies receive.**

TEXT BOOKS

Several major medical textbooks were reviewed by the working party to assess their content in respect of SCD and thalassaemia. Most texts devoted 3 – 5 pages on the pathophysiology and clinical manifestations. There was **little discussion about the treatment and management of the commonest problem in SCD, which is the painful crises**. Most texts comment that analgesia is required but do not discuss in practical terms what the doctor in A&E needs to know in everyday practice. Most nursing textbooks also do not deal with practical aspects of SCD management. Some nursing texts make little or no reference to SCD or thalassaemia. However there are rare exceptions in the case of paediatric nursing reference books, some of which deal thoroughly with the topic.

Management of the uncommon SCD emergencies is covered quite well but these only make up a small proportion of admissions most of which are for painful crises. There is little reference to counselling except that related to antenatal diagnosis.

POSTGRADUATE EDUCATION

Postgraduate medical training may need to include further education about haemoglobinopathies. Obviously this is essential for all haematologists but in parts of the country where these haematological emergencies are common it is suggested that a short **course of special instruction should be included in the 'induction course'** which is almost universal for doctors joining hospitals as SHOs or Registrars. This might be reinforced by a **'procedures' book in the A&E Department**. Aspects of haemoglobinopathy care are important for other specialties such as anaesthetists and obstetricians. It might also be a significant part of **GP postgraduate training** in an area where there are a large number of people at risk of haemoglobinopathy. More detail about clinical manifestations and management of haemoglobinopathies is available in specialist haematology text books devoted exclusively to the subject (*Ref 64, 65*), as well as monographs (*Ref 66*).

OTHER HEALTH PROFESSIONALS

Other health professionals who require education about haemoglobinopathies include **nurses, midwives and counsellors**. For nurses and midwives the extent of knowledge needs to be greater where ethnic groups at risk are a significant proportion of the general population. The Royal College of Nursing investigated knowledge among nurses and health visitors about SCDs and published a report in 1988 (*Ref 67*). Medical Laboratory Scientific Officers and others should be aware of the importance of low MCH in the context of haemoglobinopathies. Such findings should be brought to the attention of the clinicians looking after the patient.

LOCAL AUTHORITIES AND STATUTORY BODIES

Local authorities need to be aware of haemoglobinopathies in **planning their services**. This is particularly relevant in respect of responsibilities for **education, social work and housing**. There is a role here for counsellors, who may themselves be funded by local authorities. Other statutory authorities such as the **police and immigration officials** also need to be aware so as to handle situations sensitively. **Employers** both public and private need to know about haemoglobinopathies so that due allowance can be made for time off work for sickness, hospital appointments, etc.

RECOMMENDATIONS

- *District Directors of Public Health and FHSAs could increase public awareness via health promotion in GP practices, for example, by providing posters, leaflets, etc.*

- *Medical undergraduates should have educational objectives for the haemoglobinopathies.*

- *Medical undergraduates need to know about diagnosis of patients and carriers, be aware of the groups at risk, how the disorders are inherited and what treatments patients with haemoglobinopathy receive.*

- *Haemoglobinopathies should be included in vocational training, e.g. GP, obstetrics, anaesthesia etc.*

- *A permanent resource of national educational material on haemoglobinopathies is desirable.*

- *Material for patients should use appropriate words and language.*

The importance of patients having some sort of identification stating that they have a haemoglobinopathy has been referred to previously in this report. When a patient presents to an A&E Department where he is not known to the staff on duty the **possession of a haemoglobinopathy card can be most useful in promoting rapid assessment and treatment, particularly in the case of pain relief.**

HAEMOGLOBINOPATHY CARDS

In 1988 a national haemoglobinopathy card was launched by the DHSS (*Ref 68*). A multilingual explanatory leaflet was issued to accompany the card (Appendix 10). While the concept was welcomed, there was criticism of specific details (*Ref 69*). Some hospitals have produced local alternative cards.

The working party recommends that the national haemoglobinopathy card should be improved. There should be one distinctive patient-held card for all major haemoglobinopathies. A poster campaign in all A&E Departments and GP surgeries should accompany the launch of a new card in order to make it nationally recognisable. Ideally it would be a credit card-sized photocard with a named hospital contact. People with SCD arriving in A&E Departments in painful crisis could show the card to facilitate appropriate treatment. People with thalassaemia could show the card if they needed treatment in a hospital other than their usual one. One purpose of the original card (which had three versions, disease, trait or neither) was to avoid the need for retesting individuals.

PATIENT REGISTERS

There is no national register of patients with SCD, though some districts and regions have registers. A national register of people with thalassaemia was started in 1990, and figures up to 1987 are probably quite reliable (affected children may not present for 2 – 3 years). A national register of antenatal diagnosis for haemoglobinopathy disorders has recently been started. It is based on collaboration of the only 3 diagnostic laboratories involved, and figures are complete since 1974, when antenatal diagnosis first became possible.

Local confidential registers are used by some hospitals to help maintain consistency and to plan future treatment for individual patients. On such registers individuals need to be identified. National or regional registers which are helpful in determining overall planning needs require only numbers of patients and not individual data.

RECOMMENDATIONS

- *The national haemoglobinopathy card should be improved. There should be one distinctive patient-held card for all haemoglobinopathies. A thorough review should be undertaken before decisions are made.*

- *People with a haemoglobinopathy, and carriers, should be encouraged to carry haemoglobinopathy cards and those who have been tested and are negative for haemoglobinopathy should carry written evidence of this.*

- *Local registers at the relevant hospital should give full details regarding individual patients while overall numbers should be made available Regionally and Nationally for planning health care.*

SECTION 11 • MEASUREMENT OF OUTCOME

Health outcomes are the health results of illness, or of treatment for illness, while health services outcomes are all the results (not just in terms of health) of preventive or therapeutic interventions. The crude measures of morbidity and mortality may not be sophisticated enough in the case of the complex situations of patients with haemoglobinopathy, each aspect of the condition which has been considered in this report lends itself to individual detailed analysis. Deficiencies need to be recognised and agendas set to bring management up to best practice levels and the audit cycle completed by reassessment at a planned later date.

The distinction between different types of health outcomes helped us to arrange our recommendations about the measurement of outcomes under three overlapping headings:

1. Knowing more about health outcomes of haemoglobinopathies
2. Knowing more about the various effects of different interventions for people with haemoglobinopathy
3. Ensuring that services for people with haemoglobinopathy are delivered as well as possible.

1. *Knowing more about the outcomes of haemoglobinopathies*

Not enough is known by health service professionals about how the health and the quality of life of people with haemoglobinopathy are affected by their disorder and by the interventions they are offered. In the future, there should be greater concentration on the patient's experience, on health outcomes as assessed by patients, as well as health professionals.

2. *Knowing more about the various effects of different interventions for people with haemoglobinopathies.*

Time and again in the Working Party's discussions, we realised that we lacked unbiased estimates of the impact of different treatments and services for people with haemoglobinopathies: whether in terms of cost effectiveness, equity or humanity of care. This highlighted the importance of evaluative research, or what is increasingly being called "health technology assessment."

One source of information of this kind is randomised controlled trials and a list of 30 haemoglobinopathy trials published since 1983 is reproduced in Appendix 11. This list helps to identify a series of proven benefit (or of proven uselessness) and raises the question how far these trials' results have been put into practice. It also highlights the small degree to which services offered to people with haemoglobinopathy have been vigorously evaluated. So little reliable information about evaluation is available that we risk being paralysed by inaction. Put simply, if we had restricted our recommendations to those supported by controlled evaluations, we would have had little to recommend.

A way forward was suggested by the recent paper prepared by the Advisory Group Health Technology Assessment for the Director of Research and Development and published by the Department of Health (*Ref 70*) suggests: "It would be fair to meet the cost of providing forms of care which have been adopted but remain unevaluated on a standard basis, whether or not they are being offered within a research project. But the cost of providing unevaluated new forms of care within the NHS should be met only if they are being offered within the context of properly designed research to assess their effects." (Paragraph 82 of the report). We support this principle and make recommendations accordingly.

3. Ensuring that services for people with haemoglobinopathy are delivered as well as possible.
This is the task of clinical audit. The Working Party received little evidence abut the extent or impact of clinical audit in this area, but recommends that audit be pursued and developed. We speak of "clinical" rather than "medical" audit because, as the rest of our report makes clear, we are strongly committed to multi-disciplinary care of people with haemoglobinopathy. For the same reason, we believe that clinical audit will at times be superseded by multi-agency audit.

The recommendations made in this report are suitable topics for audit, particularly those with a major impact on patients' health or on cost, or those supported by experimental evidence (see Appendix 11).

Patient complaints must be taken seriously and the working party considered that questionnaires for people with haemoglobinopathies would be a useful tool in checking for patient satisfaction.

Every aspect of haemoglobinopathies considered in this report lends itself to individual detailed analysis. Examples of areas which might be evaluated are given in the table below, classified broadly in terms of aim, process and outcome.

Table 6 : Examples of areas which could be evaluated
SCREENING

AIM
- ❏ Acquire knowledge of ethnic mix of population to develop screening
- ❏ Existence of appropriate screening programme / protocol

PROCESS
- ❏ Systems to ensure specificity, sensitivity and reliability of information
- ❏ Check patient understanding of information
- ❏ Timing of screening to be appropriate
- ❏ Number of antenatal diagnoses requested, and their outcomes

OUTCOME
- ❏ Proportion of babies with SCD born in the district / region, who were detected at birth
- ❏ Proportion of couples at risk identified in time for informed reproductive choice
- ❏ Number of affected babies born without the parent's risk having been identified and genetic counselling provided (= unexpected affected births)

COUNSELLING

AIM
- ❏ To ensure that individuals at risk of haemoglobinpathy or who have the disorder have access to appropriate counselling

PROCESS
- ❏ Workload of counsellors to be monitored
- ❏ Knowledge of subject by counsellors
- ❏ Appropriate language and terms
- ❏ Co-ordination with other health professionals

OUTCOME
- ❏ Patient satisfaction improved resulting in fewer complaints about, e.g. insensitivity, directive rather than non-directive counselling

SICKLE CELL DISORDER - MANAGEMENT

AIM
- ❏ Appropriate management of people with haemoglobinpathy
- ❏ Management to be integrated across departments and professions
- ❏ To determine whether treatment to take place in haemoglobinopathy centre or other hospitals

PROCESS
- ❏ Clinical audit of management
- ❏ Case conference on each death
- ❏ Joint transfer of care from paediatrician to physician at puberty
- ❏ Commuication with primary health care and the community
- ❏ Guidelines for management in A&E followed
- ❏ Local detailed register of each individual patient
- ❏ Availability of register to A&E, Haematology Department and others
- ❏ Guidelines available in A&E
- ❏ Assessment of whether a haemoglobinopathy centre is needed
- ❏ Health professionals knowledge of management of the conditions

OUTCOME
- ❏ Reduced frequency of specific complications, e.g. orthopaedic, failure of growth and puberty, reproduction
- ❏ Reduced patient complaints – delays in treatment less frequent
- ❏ Outcomes for areas other than health, e.g. employment rates, access to appropriate housing

PAIN CONTROL

AIM
- ❏ Rapid and effective control of pain in patients with crisis

PROCESS
- ❏ Individualised pain protocol
- ❏ Clinical audit
- ❏ Guidelines on pain management available in A&E

OUTCOME
- ❏ Freedom from pain – reduced fear of painful crisis

THALASSAEMIA MAJOR – specific and additional to those for SCD – please refer

INPUT / STRUCTURE
- ❏ Regular treatment to fit in with patients' social and employment activities as far as possible

PROCESS
- ❏ Setting up transfusion – staff and pumps available
- ❏ Planning transfusions in advance

OUTCOME
- ❏ Greater patient satisfaction

CHILDREN WITH HAEMOGLOBINOPATHIES

AIM
❑ Multiprofessional management

PROCESS
❑ Penicillin for children with SCD from 3 months
❑ Contact with schools
❑ Assessment for possible bone marrow transplantation
❑ Co-operation with Community Child Health Services
❑ Psychological support
❑ Joint planning of adolescent transfer

OUTCOME
❑ Greater patient/parent satisfaction
❑ Educational achievement
❑ Improvement in morbidity caused by, e.g. infection, iron overload
❑ Patient compliance with penicillin, desferrioxamine

EDUCATION

AIM
❑ Health and other professionals, patients and their families and communities to be aware of the haemoglobinopathies

PROCESS
❑ Undergraduate education
❑ Postgraduate education
❑ Health promotion
❑ Leaflets in appropriate languages
❑ Universal availability of leaflets

OUTCOME
❑ Improved awareness leading to reduced morbidity

CARDS AND REGISTERS

AIM
❑ Local information available so that health professionals do not need to retest patients before treatment – particular pertinent to patients with painful crisis in A&E
❑ Information for planning

PROCESS
❑ User-friendly card for patients and health professionals
❑ Distribution of card to : patients, carriers and individuals tested and found negative for haemoglobinopathy genes
❑ Local confidential register available to all those with a need to know
❑ Anonymised information to Regional / National register

OUTCOME
❑ More rapid access for patients to appropriate care
❑ Better planning and organisation of services nationally

District Health Authorities are responsible for assessing the needs of their resident populations and purchasing services to provide for those needs. The District Director of Public Health (DDPH) seeks professional advice according to Circular EL(91)21 (Appendix 12).

The requirements for **comprehensive care** of haemoglobinopathy patients have been mentioned in earlier parts of the report and include screening and counselling as well as treatment. Details of the contracts may vary in different districts in line with local needs. It is useful for DDPHs to look at examples of such contracts in other districts to help in drawing up their contracts. Examples are held by the Working Party Secretariat (*Ref 71 – 73*). Funding issues should be identified and contracts need to ensure that all the necessary aspects are covered and that different aspects of care are not separated more than necessary.

HAEMOGLOBINOPATHY CENTRES

The working party recommends that **haemoglobinopathy centres should be identified in areas where there are high numbers of people with haemoglobinopathies**. WHO guidance suggests that above a threshold of 40 patients with thalassaemia major and 100 with SCD it is worthwhile having a haemoglobinopathy centre. The Working Party believes that patients would be prepared to travel to centres for regular visits. It is acknowledged that it would be difficult to demonstrate that haemoglobinopathy centres are the **best places for patient care**. Some of the advantages and disadvantages of specialist treatment centres are listed in Table 7. Centres can only realistically be established in areas where haemoglobinopathies are common. In areas with smaller numbers of the groups at risk specific **hospitals and clinicians usually develop expertise and develop routine care**. It is suggested that specialist centres with high expertise can provide a regular consultation and back-up service for other treatment centres, for example, by providing yearly or 2-yearly patient review and management back-up. Consideration of provision of services might be addressed by a **multidisciplinary working group**, which might be appropriate in such districts. This could consist of a haematologist, paediatrician, counsellor, GP, health visitor, obstetrician, midwife, public health specialist, patient representative. The Working Party was concerned that in the fluctuating situation of GP fundholding some patients may fall outside planning arrangements because tertiary referrals might be used rather than providing planned joint comprehensive care, written into contracts. This is an area which should be addressed by the multidisciplinary working group.

RECOMMENDATIONS

- *Purchasers should assess the need for haemoglobinopathy services for their resident population. Those with a high proportion of ethnic minorities at risk of haemoglobinopathy should consider commissioning comprehensive centres from provider units.*

- *Purchasers should take professional advice as recommended by the 1991 Circular (EL(91)21) when making decisions about contracting for services for the haemoglobinopathies.*

- *In placing contracts purchasers should ensure that each patient has access to comprehensive care for the condition.*

- *In comprehensive centres there should be designated beds and clinical nurse specialists, and counsellors should be part of the team looking after the patients in hospital.*

- *A multidisciplinary working group on this topic should be set up at Regional or District level depending on the numbers of people in ethnic minorities at risk of haemoglobinopathies in the populations they serve.*

- *Wherever possible patients' wishes should be taken into account when deciding where their treatment should take place.*

- *Purchasers should take account of district boundaries when contracting for services to ensure co-ordination of counselling services and treatment because counselling services are sometimes purchased separately.*

Table 7. Relative merits of general hospitals and special treatment centres for chronic disease

Place of treatment	Advantages	Common disadvantages
Specialist treatment centres	• Dedicated efficient service • Continuity of care (may include adolescents and adults) • Most up-to-date practice • Social support (meet other families) • Contact with Support Association • Psychological support • 24-hour direct telephone contact	• Distance : cost of travelling in time and money to the family • Difficulties in dealing with emergencies
General Hospital	• Closeness and convenience for family • Rapid access in emergency • More medical and nursing staff gain experience with the condition	• Isolation of family • 'End of queue' mentality • Care often delegated to junior staff • Late introduction of new treatments • Inexperience with complications, especially in adolescent patients • Lack of psychological and social support

Evidence submitted to the working party, as well as the working party's deliberations, have highlighted patients' interest in research on haemoglobinopathies and possible future advances. It is important that clinicians looking after patients with haemoglobinopathies have close contact with those in basic science research to ensure that research is targetted at those aspects which are of greatest concern to patients.

ANTI-SICKLING AGENTS

There is an **urgent need for anti-sickling agents** to prevent or shorten sickle cell crises, especially in patients with severe disorders. Approaches currently being explored to inhibit intravascular sickling may broadly be divided into (1) agents that might inhibit the gelation of haemoglobin S that occurs when it is deoxygenated, (2) agents that might modify the red cell membrane and render the cell less prone to sickling, and (3) agents to improve peripheral blood flow. Further details are given in Appendix 13.

The most promising changes thus far are the substituted benzaldehyde (589C80), hydroxyurea and cetiedil but further toxicity and clinical studies will be required before general clinical use can be considered. A drug is unlikely to be available within five years.

Butyric acid has given promising results by increasing the fetal haemoglobin level and so preventing sickling.

GENE THERAPY

The **haemoglobinopathies** were the first monogenic disorders characterised at the molecular level and so were **good candidates for gene therapy**. There have however been major difficulties. To achieve a lasting result, 'correct' genes must be inserted into haemopoietic stem cells, but these have proved very hard to identify. In addition, there is no evidence that repaired (transfected) stem cells would proliferate in preference to non-transfected haemopoietic stem cells. There is also the problem of making sure that enough normal haemoglobin is produced and ensuring synthesis of alpha and beta globin chains. As a result, interest has turned to genes where a small increase in enzyme activity may make a major difference: examples include severe combined immunodeficiency, ADA deficiency and Lesch-Nyhan Syndrome. The first, so far successful, attempt at gene therapy has been in a patient with ADA deficiency.

Ethical issues also need to be considered in relation to gene therapy, as individuals have very different views and it is a form of therapy which may be **unacceptable to some**. An expert committee, the Clothier Committee, has considered gene therapy and its report has been accepted by Ministers. The committee concluded that in appropriate circumstances, genes may be inserted into somatic cells, that is any body cell other than a germ cell. Any genetic change is confined to the altered cell population in that single recipient. Germ-line gene therapy would create much more controversy, as it would involve introducing altered genes into fertilised eggs, and the alteration would be passed on to future generations. In many of the disorders where gene therapy is being considered **alternative treatment options** are available such as bone marrow transplantation, and these may currently be considered preferable (*Ref 74 – 76*).

BONE MARROW TRANSPLANTATION (BMT)

THALASSAEMIA

Recent clinical investigation has indicated the value of **BMT** in haemoglobinopathies. In particular, the data from Lucarelli (*Ref 54*) indicate that the best treatment for **Beta thalassaemia major** is BMT in the early years of life, that is, before **iron accumulation** has caused any **organ damage** and usually before the age of 12 years. Ideally the donor should be an **immunologically matched** brother or sister who does not have thalassaemia major. Unfortunately the chances of such a match are only approximately **1 in 4**.

SICKLE CELL DISORDER

The role of **BMT** in **SCD** is less well established (*Ref 77*). It is not possible to predict the 10 – 20% of patients with SCD who will have severe crises and complications. Current data suggests that BMT should be considered when a child is young and when the prediction of the severity of the disorder is least certain. It is therefore difficult to justify such a procedure with a **mortality of some 5 – 10%** for a child who might otherwise have been substantially unaffected. As methods of predicting severity of SCD improve as well as BMT techniques, it seems possible that BMT could become the treatment of choice for SCD unless an effective, safe, anti-sickling drug becomes available in the meantime.

ORAL IRON CHELATING AGENTS

There is a long history of efforts to find a satisfactory oral iron chelator. This would help **compliance with treatment**, as a significant number of patients with thalassaemia major have difficulty in maintaining regular treatment with parenteral desferrioxamine.

It is hoped that the cost of chelation treatment might also fall as a result of using an oral iron chelator. Although some compounds have reached clinical trials, at present there is no indication of when a safe and effective compound will become available.

ANTENATAL DIAGNOSIS

NEW TECHNIQUES

PRE-IMPLANTATION DIAGNOSIS

Many couples at risk express the wish to be able to **start pregnancy** knowing the **baby** would be **unaffected**. It now seems a **realistic possibility** to develop methods of **pre-implantation diagnosis** by combining the new ultra-sensitive DNA technology with *in vitro* fertilisation (IVF) techniques. However, **many difficulties must still be overcome**, for example, the risk of mis-diagnosis due to contamination with even a single human cell and the limited success in establishing pregnancy following IVF.

ANTENATAL DIAGNOSIS USING FETAL CELLS OBTAINED FROM THE MATERNAL BLOOD

There is now good evidence that a small number of cells originating from the placenta can be extracted from a sample of the mother's blood in **early pregnancy**. In some cases genetic diagnosis may be possible using these cells so there is hope that a **non-invasive and therefore risk free approach** could be developed. However, for a reliable diagnosis the provisional diagnosis on cells so obtained would need to be **confirmed by conventional antenatal diagnosis** methods. The approach could be particularly useful for couples who refuse antenatal testing because of the associated obstetric risk.

OTHER RESEARCH NEEDS

Studies of outcome following specific interventions are in **short supply** and careful studies are needed in order to inform purchasers of the best means of providing **comprehensive care for haemoglobinopathy patients to reduce morbidity and mortality and to promote health and well-being**.

The Medical Research Council (MRC) and the Overseas Development Agency have funded the MRC Laboratories in Jamaica for over 20 years. Cohorts of patients with SCD have been studied over this period to assess the natural history of the disorder and the effects of interventions. Similar **cohorts are now being followed in the UK, where the pattern of complications differs,** e.g. painful crises are more common in the UK and leg ulcers are more common in Jamaica. The Working Party considers that extension of UK-based **clinical and epidemiological research should be funded by the MRC**. It was suggested that approaches also be made to the central Research and Development Directorate at the Department of Health as well as to Regional Directors of Research and Development.

RECOMMENDATIONS

- *Clinicians should keep abreast of new developments and introduce them after proper evaluation has been undertaken.*

- *There should be carefully controlled development in bone marrow transplantation for SCD.*

- *Anti-sickling agents should be considered when further research and clinical trials demonstrate their efficiency.*

- *Further research should be conducted into use of oral iron chelating agents.*

- *New research developments for haemoglobinopathies should be supported.*

SECTION 14 : RECOMMENDATIONS

These are a summary of recommendations but more specific recommendations are given in the specific sections.

PURCHASERS OF HEALTH CARE

- Purchasers should assess the need for haemoglobinopathy services for their resident population. Those with a high proportion of ethnic minorities at risk of haemoglobinopathy should consider commissioning comprehensive centres from provider units.

- Purchasers should take professional advice as recommended by the 1991 Circular (EL(91)21) when making decisions about contracting for services for the haemoglobinopathies.

- In placing contracts purchasers should ensure that each patient has access to comprehensive care for the condition.

- In comprehensive centres there should be designated beds and clinical nurse specialists, and counsellors should be part of the team looking after the patient in hospital.

- A multi disciplinary working group on this topic should be set up at Regional or District level depending on the numbers of people in ethnic minorities at risk of haemoglobinopathies in the populations they serve.

- Wherever possible patients' wishes should be taken into account when deciding where their treatment should take place.

- Purchasers should take account of district boundaries when contracting for services to ensure co-ordination of counselling services and treatment because counselling services are sometimes purchased separately

- Local registers at the relevant hospital should give full details regarding individual patients while overall numbers should be made available Regionally and Nationally for planning health care.

REGIONS

- Every Regional Director of Public Health has a role for ensuring that purchasers demand the relevant screening and appropriate counselling.

PROVIDERS OF TREATMENT

- An identified clinician, with a nominated deputy, should have responsibility for overall patient care.

- All staff involved with haemoglobinopathies should be trained in giving accurate information. Providers should ensure that health professionals, midwives, for example, are adequately trained before undertaking non-directive counselling.

- Treatment needs to be organised to minimise disturbance of patients' daily lives as much as possible.

- Forward planning of patients' admissions should ensure that delays in setting up transfusions are avoided if at all possible. Patients should be provided with explanations for delay if it occurs.

Pain relief

- Pain relief should be fast and adequate and monitored by trained staff. A pain management protocol is necessary in hospitals which treat patients in sickle cell crisis and is essential in specialist haemoglobinopathy units.

- Guidelines for the management of acute sickle cell crises should be available and prominently displayed in every A&E.department. These guidelines should have been prepared in co-operation with the relevant departments, e.g. haematology, paediatrics and A&E itself and should cover the rapid relief of acute pain and the management of precipitating factors and life threatening complications.

- If patients are known or carrying a haemoglobinopathy card they should be treated immediately with the drug shown on the card if it is apparent to the receiving physician that they are having a crisis or starting one. If patients are not known or not carrying a card they should be given Entonox or a single dose of a strong analgesic until further information indicates that they are having a sickle cell crisis.

- The patient and the hospital consultant should mutually agree which analgesic the patient may require for an acute crisis. Adequate information should be available to the patient with regard to drug potency, side effects and problems of accumulation and metabolites. The name of this drug and its dose and route of administration should be given on the haemoglobinopathy card and on the patient's records.

- Each patient should have an individual plan for the management of pain. Individuals should be given enough information to make informed decisions about their choice of drug.

- Entonox is a useful analgesic for use in ambulances and A&E. It should not be used at home.

For children additionally

- Children with SCD should have **prophylactic penicillin** from not later than 3 months old in addition to vaccination against pneumoccocus

- Patients should be managed jointly by paediatricians and haematologists and the transfer at adolescence should be jointly planned.

- Where possible there should be a facility for direct admission to a designated children's ward.

- Facilities should be available for parents to stay overnight with their children.

- All children should be registered with a haemoglobinopathy centre.

GPs (PROVIDERS OF PRIMARY CARE)

- There should be good communication between the hospital consultants and GPs in the area to provide continuity of care. There is merit in FHSAs recognising a few GPs and their practices to take special interest in the primary care management of those patients with haemoglobinopathies in coroperation with specialist services.

- All GPs with significant numbers of the relevant ethnic groups on their lists should be encouraged to take part in haemoglobinopathy screening.

- Preconceptional carrier diagnosis should be encouraged and GPs have a significant part to play in this.

- FHSAs should suggest GPs to include assessment of risk of haemoglobinopathy in new patients joining their practices.

- In acute crisis, patients may be give short acting oral morphine by GPs because it is reversible.

- The GP has a role in the management of chronic pain, for example, for patients with avascular hip necrosis, and also in the provision of self-administered analgesic for early crisis management.

- Partial agonist and antagonist opioid drugs eg buprenorphine, pentazocine, are not recommended for treatment of acute pain before transfer to hospital, eg, by the GP.

SCREENING SERVICES

- All patients from ethnic minorities at risk of SCD should be screened pre-operatively unless written records show this has been done already.

- If there is any doubt whether the mother or the father of the child is at risk of haemoglobinopathy the individual should be screened.

- Individuals should be informed if they are being tested, their names recorded and they should be informed of the result in writing whether it is **positive or negative**.

- Preconceptional carrier diagnosis should be encouraged and GPs have a significant part to play in this.

- A co-ordinated antenatal screening programme, including the haemoglobinopathies, should be supported.

- If the population coming through the antenatal clinic is composed of 15% or more ethnic minorities at risk of SCD, there should be universal antenatal screening (ideally before 10 weeks into pregnancy) and neonatal screening. In other circumstances selective screening should be targeted appropriately.

- The Guthrie card and the capillary method are equally good methods for neonatal screening.

- Cord blood samples should be avoided for neonatal screening.

COUNSELLING SERVICES

- Haemoglobinopathy counsellors should be available in sufficient numbers to ensure that the needs of both primary health care and hospitals are met.

- Designated counsellors should be properly trained and the counselling service must be co-ordinated with other aspects of the management of the haemoglobinopathies. In areas with small numbers of people at risk this work may be combined with other responsibilities.

- Counsellors should speak appropriate languages, wherever possible.

- Counsellors should assist self help groups to provide help for affected families in the community.

GOVERNMENT AGENCIES AND DEPARTMENTS AND RESEARCH BODIES

- The national haemoglobinopathy card should be improved. There should be one distinctive patient held card for all haemoglobinopathies. A thorough review should be undertaken before decisions are made.

- Research is needed to determine at what frequency of population at risk of haemoglobinopathy it is appropriate to do universal neonatal screening.

- Research is needed particularly in the area of screening for SCD and thalassaemia to determine how decisions are made about testing, and the effects of being tested and declining testing.

- Research is needed into the most effective and appropriate methods of delivering haemoglobinopathy counselling services.

- There should be carefully controlled development in bone marrow transplantation for SCD.

- Anti-sickling agents should be considered when further research and clinical trials demonstrate their efficiency.

- Further research should be conducted into the use of oral iron chelating agents.

- Randomised clinical trials are needed to test the relative value of pethidine and morphine and new drugs.

ALL THOSE RESPONSIBLE FOR EDUCATIONAL ACTIVITIES

- Medical undergraduates should have educational objectives for the haemoglobinopathies.

- Medical undergraduates need to know about diagnosis of patients and carriers, be aware of the groups at risk, how the disorders are inherited and what treatments patients with haemoglobinopathies receive.

- Haemoglobinopathies should be included in vocational training, eg, GP, obstetric, anaesthesia etc

- District Directors of Public Health and FHSAs could increase public awareness via health promotion in GP practices, for example, by providing posters, leaflets, etc.

- Clinicians should keep abreast of new developments and introduce them after proper evaluation has been undertaken.

- All those linked with the care of children with haemoglobinopathies (including parents, teachers and health professionals) need to be made aware of these conditions and the requirements of children who have them.

- A permanent resource of national educational material on haemoglobinopathies is desirable.

- Material for patients should use appropriate words and language.

PATIENTS AND PATIENT GROUPS

- The patient and the hospital consultant should mutually agree which analgesic the patient may require for an acute crisis. Adequate information should be available to the patient with regard to drug potency, side effects and problems of accumulation and metabolites. The name of this drug and its dose should be given on the haemoglobinopathy card and on the patient's records.

- People with a haemoglobinopathy and carriers should be encouraged to carry haemoglobinopathy cards and those who have been tested and are negative for haemoglobinopathy should carry written evidence of this.

- Counsellors should assist self help groups to provide help for affected families in the community.

REFERENCES

1. Pain in Sickle Cell Disease: Setting standards of care
The proceedings of a one-day conference held on 19th September, 1991, in the University of Wales College of Medicine, Cardiff, Wales on behalf of STAC – the Sickle Cell and Thalassaemia Association of Counsellors. Shankleman, J and A May Eds. Published by the Community Health Unit, SGHA 1993.

2. The Haemoglobinopathies in Europe: Combined report on two WHO meetings. 1988.

3. Social and genetic implications of customary consanguineous marriage among British Pakistanis: Galton Institute Occasional Papers, Second Series, No 4. 1992.

4. OPCS 1991 Census Coding Frame

5. NHSME Dear Colleague Letter – Collection of Information on Patients Ethnic Group – dated 9 July 1992.

6. Haemoglobinopathy Screening: Prepared by the General Haematology Task Force: Edited by B Roberts on behalf of the British Committee for Standards in Haematology. Clinical and Laboratory Haematology 10:87–94. 1988.

7. Holland W W. Screening : reasons to be cautious BMJ 306 : 1222 – 3 1993

8. Wilson J M G, Jungner G. Principles and practice of screening for disease. Geneva : World Health Organisation, 1968

9. Guidelines for Prenatal Diagnosis of Haemoglobinopathies: Prepared by Working Party of BCSH General Haematology Task Force. (1993) Submitted for publication

10. Guidelines for the Investigation of the Thalassaemia Traits: Prepared by Working Party to BCSH General Haematology Task Force. (1993) Submitted for publication

11. Anionwu E, Patel N, Kanji G et al. Counselling for prenatal diagnosis of sickle cell disease and beta thalassaemia major. A four year experience: J Medical Genetics, 25:769 – 772. 1988.

12. Moisley C, Modell B, McKeigue P M, et al. Use of a patient register for evaluating delivery of screening and genetic counselling for thalassaemia in the UK.

13. Green, J M & France-Dawson, M 1993. Women's experiences of routine screening during pregnancy: the sickle cell study. In Targetting Health Promotion: Reaching Those In Need. Proceedings of a symposium. Published by the Health Promotion Research Trust, Cambridge.

14. Milne R. Assessment of care of children with sickle cell disease: implications for neonatal screening programmes. BMJ 300:371– 4. 1990.

15. Foshlock K, Henderson S, Bellingham A J. Neonatal Screening for Haemoglobinopathies in Camberwell Health District. 1989.

16. CMO Professional letter PL CMO 93 – Services for Genetic Disorders – In Press.

17. Marteau, T M. Psychological implications of prenatal diagnosis. In: Drife, Jo & Donnai D. Antenatal Diagnosis of Fetal Abnormalities. (pp 243 – 254). London: Springer-Verlag Ltd. 1991

18. Marteau T M, Slack J, Kidd J, et al. Presenting a routine screening test in antenatal care: Practice observed. Public Health 106:131–141. 1992.

19. Marteau T M, Obstetricians presenting amniocentesis to pregnant women: Practice Observed. Journal of Reproductive and Infant Psychology.

20. Royal College of Physicians . Prenatal Diagnosis and Genetic Screening. Community & Service Implications RCP London 1989.

21. Marteau T M. Psychological implications of genetic screening. In: Evers-Kiebooms, JP Fryns, JJ Cassiman, H van den Berghe (Eds). Psychological Aspects of Genetics (pp 185 – 190). New York: Wiley-Liss.

22. Stevenson A C, Davison B C C. Genetic Counselling, page 274, William Heinemann, London. 1976.

23. Psychosocial Aspects of Genetic Counselling: Proceedings of a Conference Held September 24 – 26 1990, Belgium.

24. NAHAT (1991) Words about Action: Haemoglobinopathies (Sickle Cell Disorders and Thalassaemia) Bulletin No 4 January 1991. National Association of Health.

25. Anionwu E. Survey of Haemoglobinopathy Counsellors, January 1992.

26. Guidelines for ambulance personnel when dealing with people with sickle cell anaemia or similar conditions usually grouped together as sickle cell disease: Sickle Cell Society guidelines.

27. Strategies for the Care of Patients with Sickle Cell Disease: Barts NHS Trust, 1992

28. Sickle Cell Disease – A short guide to management: Prepared by M Brozovic on behalf of the WHO/Mediterranean Working Group on Haemoglobinopathies in 1988, revised 1989.

29. Guidelines for sedation by non-anaesthetists published under the aegis of the Commission of Provision of Surgical Services. Published by the Royal College of Surgeons of England 1993

30. Brozovic M, Anionwu E. Sickle Cell Disease in Britain. J Clin Pathol 37:1321–26. 1984

31. Brozovic M, Davies S C, Brownell A I. Acute admissions of patients with sickle cell disease who live in Britain. BMJ 294 : 1987.

32. Franklin I M. Services for Sickle Cell Disease: Unified Approach Needed. BMJ Vol 296

33. Sickle Cell Disease and the Non-Specialist. Drug & Therapeutics Bulletin, Vol 27, No 3. 1989.

34. Brozovic M. Sickle Cell Disease. Prescribers' Journal Vol 32. 1992

35. Moriarty B J. Sickle Cell retinopathy : diagnosis and management. Ophthalmic dialogue

36. Moriarty B J, Webb D K, Serjeant G R. Treatment of sub-retinal neovascularisation in association with angioid streaks in sickle cell retinopathy. Archives of Ophthalmology 72 : 1327–1328. 1987

37. Ballas S K. Treatment of pain in adults with sickle cell disease. American Journal of Haematology 34:49 –54. 1990.

38. Mitchell A, Brunner M, Fisher A P, et al. Pethidine for painful crises in Sickle Cell Disease. BJA Vol 69: 233 – 235. 1992

39. Pain in Sickle Cell Disease: proceedings of a symposium held at Central Middlesex Hospital, London in 1983. A Sickle Cell Society Publication. Editor, ASJ Baughan

40. Shankel S W, Johnson D C, Clark P S et al. Acute renal failure and glomerulopathy caused by nonsteroidal anti-inflammatory drugs. Arch Intern Med Vol 152: 986 – 990.

41. Harris K. The role of prostaglandins in the control of renal function. British Journal of Anaesthethesia. Vol 69 No. 3 1992

42. Platt O S, Thorington B T, Brambilla D, et al. Pain in Sickle Cell Disease, Rates and Risk Factors. The New England Journal of Medicine Vol 325 : 11 – 16. 1991.

43. Management of acute pain: a practical guide. International Association for the Study of Pain: Task Force on Acute Pain. 1992.

44. Perttunen K, Kalso E, Heinonen J et al. I V Diclofenac in post thoracotomy pain. British Journal of Anaesthesia 68:474 – 480. 1992.

45. Pryle B J, Grech H, Stoddart P A, et al. Toxicity of Norpethidine in Sickle Cell Crises. BMJ 304:1478 – 9. 1992.

46. UK Thalassaemia Society Newsletter 1991

47. An example of a pain protocol for children: The Hospitals for Sick Children, Great Ormond Street

48. The Welfare of CHildren and Young People in Hospital. (DH Publication)

49. Sartori P C E, Gordon G J, Darbyshire P J. Continuous Paraveretum infusion for the control of pain in painful sickling crises. Archives of Disease in Childhood 65: 1151 – 1153. 1990.

50. Samuels MP, Stebbins VA, Davies SC, Picton-Jones E, Southall DP. Sleep-related upper airway obstruction and hypoxaemia in sickle cell disease. Archives of Disease in Childhood 67:925 – 929 1992

51. Davies SC, (Personal Communication)

52. Ohene-Frempong K Seminars in Haematology 28: 213 – 219. 1991

53. Vichinsky E Seminars in Haematology   28: 220 – 226. 1991

54. Lucarelli G, Galimberti M, Polchi P, et al. Bone Marrow Transplantation in patients with Thalassaemia. N Eng J Med 322: 417 – 21. 1990

55. Evans, D. Bone Marrow Transplantation for Thalassaemia Major. J Clin Pathol 45: 553 – 555. 1992

56. Alpha Zero Thalassaemia Trait: Perinatal Centre, Department of Obstetrics and Gynaecology, University College Hospital.

57. Prenatal Diagnosis for Thalassaemia Major: Perinatal Centre, Dept of Obstetrics and Gynaecology, University College Hospital.

58. Information for People who carry Alpha Thalassaemia Trait: Perinatal Centre, Dept of Obstetrics and Gynaecology, University College Hospital.

59. Anionwu E and Jibril H (1986) A Handbook on Sickle Cell Disease: A Guide for Families. A Sickle Cell Society publication.

60. All you need to know about Thalassaemia Trait: A UK Thalassaemia Society Publication.

61. Is Sickle Cell or Thalassaemia your child's inheritance? Produced by INHOUSE Public Relations, NETRHA.

62. Greek self help package: held by the Secretariat.

63. Modell B, Vullo R. What is Thalassaemia? Thalassaemia International Federation. 1990

64. Serjeant E R. Sickle Cell Disease. 2nd edition. Oxford University Press 1992

65. Wetherall D and Clegg J B 3rd edition. Blackwell Scientific Publications 1981

66. Cao A, Gabutti V, Masera G, et al Management protocol for the Treatment of Thalassaemia Patients. Distributed by the Thalassaemia International Federation

67. France-Dawson, M. An Investigation in Sickle Cell Disorders – Nurses and Health Visitors Knowledge of the conditions, Unit Report, Daphne Heald Research Unit, RCN, London 1988.

68. Haemoglobinopathy cards: PL/CM0(88)11, PL/CN0(88)6, PL/CD0(88)1.

69. Surveys of haemoglobinopathy cards: held by Secretariat

70. Recent papers form the Advisory Group Health Technology Assessment for RDD.

71. Example of contract for haemoglobinopathies held by Secretariat.

72. Example of contract for haemoglobinopathies held by Secretariat.

73. Example of contract for haemoglobinopathies held by Secretariat.

74. Weatherall, D. Gene Therapy. BMJ 298 : 691–3. 1989

75. Weatherall, D J. Gene Therapy in Perspective. Nature. 349 : 275–76 1991

76. Weatherall, D. Current Controversies and New Horizons. Gene Therapy. Organ Transplantation: current clinical and immunological concepts. 155–65 Bailline Tindall 1989

77. Smith, R. Using a mock trial to make a difficult clinical decision. BMJ 305:1284 –7. 1992

APPENDICES

1. Individuals and groups who submitted evidence to the Working Party.

2. Sickle Cell Disorder and Thalassaemia Campaign National Demands.

3. Figures of incidence, birth rate and inheritance of haemoglobinopathies in the UK.

4. Table of Weeks pregnant at first Booking. (Sickle Cell Study).

5. Confidential Enquiry into Counselling for Genetic Disorders.

6. Number of counsellors compared with work load.

7. Summary of Recommendations for Management of Major Thalassaemia Syndromes. (Thalassaemia International Federation)

8. Psychological Support for Patients with Thalassaemia. (Thalassaemia International Federation)

9. Presentation of Child in Pain with SCD – GOS protocol

10. Haemoglobinopathy Card and leaflet. (DHSS 1988)

11. Haemoglobinopathy trials.

12. EL (91) 21

13. Anti Sickling Agents – Summary of current status.

APPENDIX 1 – Individuals and Groups who submitted evidence

Action for Sick Children

African Family Advisory Service (at Save the Children)

Association of Clinical Pathologists

Association of Community Health Councils for England and Wales

Barts NHS Trust, Department of Nursing and Quality Assurance and Department of Haematology

Birmingham Family Health Services Authority

British Paediatric Association

British Society for Haematology

Bristol Sickle Cell and Thalassaemia Centre

Charalampous , Mr. A

College of Ophthalmologists

Confederation of Indian Organisations (UK)

Dewsbury Health Authority

East Anglian Regional Health Authority

East Birmingham District Health Authority

East Oxford Health Authority

East Oxford Health Centre

East Surrey Health Authority

Garnet, Mrs C

Greater London Association of Community Health Councils

Greenwich Race an Health Project

Hastings Health Authority

Health Education Authority

Health Visitor's Association

Hospitals for Sick Children, Great Ormond Street

Isle of Man Government

King's Fund Centre for Health Services Development

Lambeth Sickle Cell and Thalassaemia Centre

Leicester Health Authority

Luton and Dunstable Hospital

Malkarni, Mrs

Marteau, Dr. T

Maternity Alliance

Mersey Regional Health Authority

Natinal Community Health Resource

National Perinatal Epidemiology Unit

North East Thames Regional Health Authority

North Western Regional Health Authority

Northern Regional Health Authority

Organisation for Sickle Cell Anaemia Research (UK)

Overseas Doctor's Association in the UK Limited

Oxford Regional Health Authority

Oxford Regional Pain Relief Unit

Preston Health Authority

Royal College of General Practitioners

Royal College of Midwifery

Royal College of Nursing of the United Kingdom

Royal College of Obstetricians and Gynaecologists

Royal College of Physicians, Faculty of Occupational Medicine

Royal College of Psychiatrists

Royal College of Radiologists

Royal College of Surgeons

Save the Children

South East London Comissioning Authority

Sickle Cell and Thalassaemia Association of Counsellors

Sickle Cell Society

South Bedfordshire Health Authority

South Birmingham District Health Authority

South East Thames Regional Health Authority

South Western Regional Health Authority

States of Guernsey Board of Health, Community Health Department

Trent Regional Health Authority

UK Thalassaemia Society

University College and Middlesex School of Medicine

Voluntary Organisations Liaison Council for Under Fives

Watford Sickle Cell Support Group

Weatherall, Professor Sir David

Welsh Office

Wessex Regional Health Authority

West Birmingham Community Care (NHS) Trust

West Midlands Regional Health Authority

Wexham Park Hospital

Whittington and Royal Northern Hospitals

Wonke, Dr. B

Yorkshire Regional Health Authority

SICKLE CELL DISORDER AND THALASSAEMIA CAMPAIGN NATIONAL DEMANDS

SICKLE CELL DISORDER AND THALASSAEMIA CAMPAIGN NATIONAL DEMANDS

1. PAIN CONTROL

Protocols should be drawn up that describe the medication and techniques available for the relief of pain, the characteristics of each and when pain control teams should be involved.

People with Sickle Cell Disorders should not have pain relief witheld while they are waiting for a full medical examination in Casualty or because they are waiting for admission to a ward.

Pain relief for inpatients should not be witheld because of staff shortages and poor organisation of the nursing and medical staff.

2. RESEARCH

The Medical Research Council should have sickle cell disorders and thalassaemia as research priorities and to start with should initiate projects to investigate the means by which sickling crises can be reversed and pain controlled more effectively.

3. SCREENING OF NEWBORNS AND COUNSELLING

There should be a national policy on screening of newborns in order that preventive measures can be undertaken shortly after birth. Screening should not be left to the discretion of the District Health Authority. Clear instructions should be given to District Health Authorities to provide screening of all newborns (using the Guthrie cards) or selective screening according to the size of the population at risk. These instructions should take into account that people do not always use services within their own District. Counselling of families and follow-up of children diagnosed as having sickle cell disorders or thalassaemia must be provided as part of the screening programme.

4. USERS FORUM

Government funding should be made available to voluntary organisations in each health district to encourage the establishment of User Forums to enable people with sickle cell disorders and thalassaemia to provide a user's perspective on the health authority's service.

5. HEALTH PROFESSIONALS

GPs should receive training in the control of pain, the nature of sickle cell crises and the need for screening of newborn babies, parents and others from the at-risk population, accompanied by counselling.

Education on sickle cell disorders should be included in the pre- and post-registration training and in-service training of all health professionals.

National medical and nursing guidelines should be devised for staff on the management of patients with sickle cell disorders and thalassaemia and the evaluation of the care which they give.

6. INFORMATION, EDUCATION AND TRAINING

Funding should be identified and made available for a comprehensive education programme. This will involve a public awareness campaign aimed at the general population, specific information for sicklers and those coping with thalassaemia and their families and carers and for those at-risk. Education about scd and thalassaemia should also be established in the curricula for health workers currently practising, and for those in voluntary organisations and local authorities.

7. SCHOOLS

Local Education Authorities should ensure that school curricula include discussion of sickle cell disorders and thalassaemia and that there are appropriate learning materials available to do this. Teachers should be trained in order that they understand the appropriate means of preventing crises and responding to children in crisis.

8. LOCAL AUTHORITIES

A National Code of Practice should be developed to guide local authorities in the provision of appropriate housing and heating for people with sickle cell disorders.

9. EMPLOYMENT

Policies should be developed through the TUC and Department of Employment, to encourage employers to show sensitivity to the needs of employees who have thalassaemia or sickle cell disorders. In particular they need to appreciate the degree of pain suffered and the reasons for admission into hospital for people with crises and the reasons for needing time off for counselling and routine clinic attendance.

The Manpower Services Commission should also provide public information for employers who are providing training for sicklers and people with thalassaemia.

10. BONE MARROW TRANSPLANTATION

There should be an equitable policy for bone marrow transplantation for people with haemoglobinopathies, so that access for people with thalassaemia and sickle cell disorders equals that of people with leukaemia and lymphoma.

This AGM urges the Department of Health to provide central support, guidance and finance to facilitate a comprehensive, equitable, appropriate and accessible service for people with sickle cell disorders (SCD) and Thalassaemia.

This AGM calls upon the Department of Health to introduce the following specific measures:

a) Universal screening of new born babies for SCD and Thalassaemia.

b) An obligation on NHS commissioning authorities to ensure that their resident population has full access to a dedicated counselling service for people with Thalassaemia, SCD or trait and in particular for:

i) people who are newly diagnosed

ii) parents of newly diagnosed babies (this should be non-directive, genetic counselling)

iii) people coping with painful crises and their social consequences

iv) people coping with the trauma of the daily use of the desferal pump required because of the need for monthly blood transfusions.

c) The development of national policies on pain control, hospital care and prevention of crises, to guide health workers who are treating people with sickle cell anaemia and Thalassaemia.

d) An education and training programme for community health workers and GPs to ensure that appropriate information, advice and counselling is offered through generic services.

e) The adoption of the Ten Point Charter (attached) devised by sickle cell and Thalassaemia organisations with CHC and other user representatives.

Proposed by: Camberwell CHC

Seconded by: Hackney CHC

Passed unanimously at GLACHC AGM 25th June 1991

THE GREATER LONDON ASSOCIATION OF COMMUNITY HEALTH COUNCILS
100 PARK VILLAGE EAST·LONDON NW1 3SR·TEL 071·387 2171
THIS ORGANISATION IS FUNDED BY LONDON BOROUGHS GRANTS COMMITTEE

APPENDIX 3 : Figures of incidence, birth rate and inheritance of haemoglobinopathies and some other major inherited disorders in the UK.

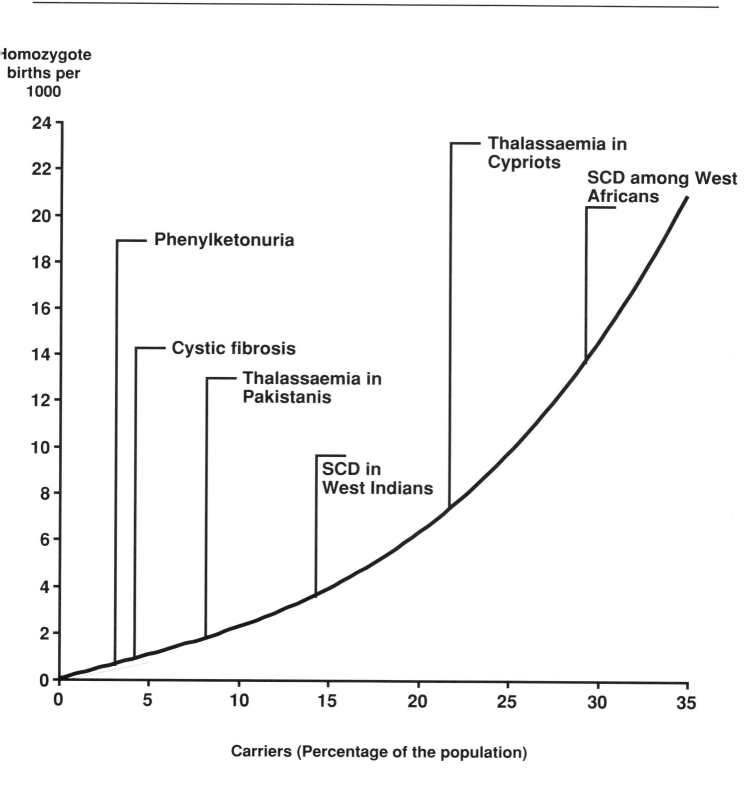

Figure 1 : Relationship between the birth-rate of homozygotes with recessively-inherited conditions and carrier frequency

Figure 2 : Recessive inheritance

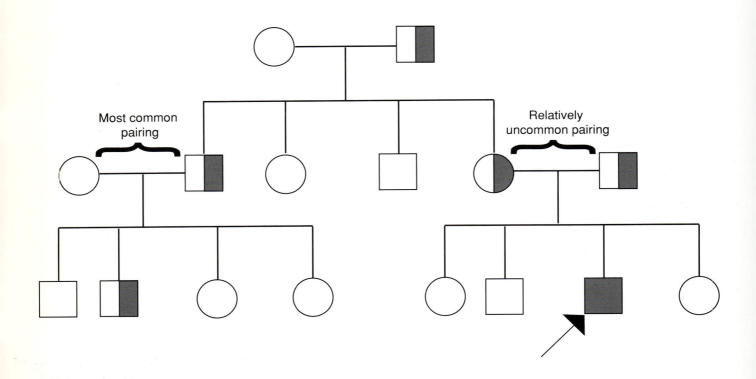

Most common pairing

Relatively uncommon pairing

☐ **Male**

◯ **Female**

▨ **Abnormal gene**

➤ **Affected individuals**

Table 1 : Table of Incidence of Haemoglobinopathies in different ethnic groups in the United Kingdom

| Ethnic group | β-thal | % of group carrying | | | | "Homozygotes"[1] | |
		α[1]-thal	Hb E	Hb S	Hb C	Total	born / 1,000
Afro-Caribbean[2]	1.5	–	–	10	3 – 5	11 – 14	3.0 – 4.5
West African	1 – 2	0	0	20 – 25	0 – 15[3]	20 – 25	9.3 – 19.2
Indian	3 – 10	0	0	0	0	3 – 10	0.23 – 2.5
Pakistani	4 – 6	0	0	0	?	4 – 6	2.0[4]
Bangladeshi	1 – 3	0	3.0	0	0	4 – 6	0.4[4]
East African Asian	6 – 10	0	0	0	0	6 – 10	0.9 – 2.5
Cypriot	16	1 – 2	0	1	0	18	7.2
Middle Eastern	3 – 5	0	0	0	0	> 3.0	0.46[4]
Chinese	3	5 – 6	0	0	0	8	1.0

[1] Includes compound conditions such as Hb S/C disease. Hb S/B-thalassaemia etc.

[2] Figures given are for Jamaicans, one of the most thoroughly-studied groups, and one of the largest groups of Afro-Caribbeans in the UK. The figures for other groups of Afro-Caribbeans are similar

[3] Very high incidence only in certain groups, e.g. Ghanaians

[4] Corrected for effects of frequent cousin marriage

Table 2 : 1991 Census : Ethnic group by approximate[1] NHS region

Region	Census counts[2] Total census count	Ethnic groups[3]	% ethnic groups
Northern	3,026,732	38,547	1.3%
Yorkshire	3,573,894	177,869	5.0%
Trent	4,637,195	203,819	4.4%
East Anglian	2,027,004	43,395	2.1%
NW Thames	3,409,589	559,011	16.4%
NE Thames	3,693,376	513,469	13.9%
SE Thames	3,607,552	278,518	7.7%
SW Thames	2,917,306	206,083	7.1%
Wessex	2,875,761	46,060	1.6%
Oxford	2,493,124	127,795	5.1%
South Western	3,399,787	47,318	1.4%
West Midlands	5,150,187	424,363	8.2%
Mersey	2,360,258	35,281	1.5%
North Western	3,883,439	209,337	5.4%
ALL ENGLAND	47,055,204	2,910,865	6.2%
Wales	2,835,073	41,551	1.5%
ENGLAND AND WALES	49,890,277	2,952,416	5.9%

[1] Figures relate to FHSAs reporting to each Regional Health Authority
[2] No adjustment has been made for Census under numeration
[3] All persons who were not reported as "White" on the Census schedule

Table 3 : Calculated (potential) annual births of infants with major haemoglobin disorders in England and Wales (Based on 1991 Census counts of population by ethnic origin)

Ethnic groups	Number (000s)	Births[1]/ 1.000	Annual births[1]	Percent Carriers	Affected / 1,000	Annual affected births
Sickle cell group						
Black Caribbean	499	15.5	7,733	12	3.6	27
Black African	210	24.3	5,108	25	15.6	80
Black Other	176	41.7	7,334	—[2]	—[2]	53
Subtotal	885		20,175			160
Thalassaemia group						
Indian ⎰ Indian	600		10,837	3	0.23	2.5
⎱	(830)	18.1	(14,922)			} 6
E. African Asian	230		4,154	6	0.9	3.7
Pakistani	455	27.1	12,328	5	1.25[3]	15
Bangladeshi	162	30.9	5,004	5	0.41	2
Chinese	146	14.5	2,113	8	0.86	2[4]
Other Asian	193	16.3	3,149	3.5	0.3	1
Cypriots[5]	160	15.0	2,402	17	7	17
Subtotal	1,946		39,987			43

[1] Estimated as one fifth of the Census count of population aged 0 – 4, adjusted for the birth rate in England and Wales between April 1986 and March 1991.

[2] This group has been assumed to comprise the same proportion of Black Caribbean and Black African as those with stated origins.

[3] Allowance has been made for the effects of consanguineous marriage.

[4] Three quarters of Chinese affected are still-births due to alpha-thalassaemia; only one quarter are thalassaemia major.

[5] The figure for Cypriot groups are synthetic estimates based on the Labour Force Survey.

APPENDIX 4 : Frequency of weeks gestation at first booking

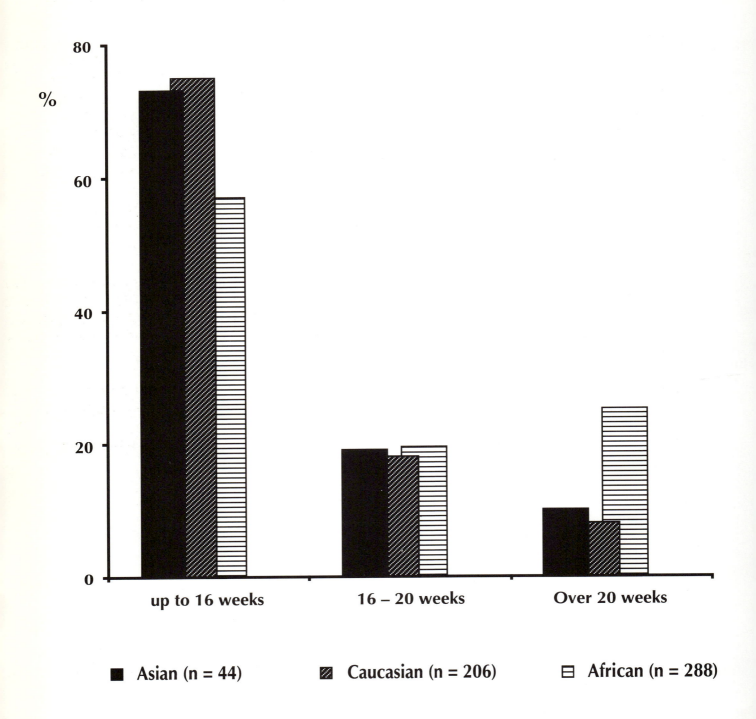

Figure 3 : Weeks pregnant at first booking. (Sickle Cell study)

APPENDIX 5 : Confidential Enquiry into Counselling for Genetic Disorders

1. This Enquiry is funded by the Department of Health as part of its clinical audit programme in collaboration with the Royal College of Physicians of London and is based in the Department of Medical Genetics, University of Manchester. It has the support of medical Royal Colleges and other professional groups, and lay organisations. The Enquiry is overseen by a Steering Committee which includes convenors who are international authorities in the disorders selected for enquiry. The purpose is to encourage greater awareness and understanding of the significance of genetics in clinical practice and its implications for services.

2. The Enquiry consists of a confidential scrutiny of recorded information of the antecedent circumstances of (i) children who are affected by selected genetic disorders, and (ii) the development in adults of selected genetic disorders, including hereditary cancers.

3. Clinicians review their own records and are encouraged to involve junior staff in this process. The means of ascertainment rely on existing registers and the professional links that have been forged by the convenors. Completed questionnaires are received and held in confidence by a co-ordinator who removes any means of identifying patients or clinicians before the data are passed to an enquiry team for analysis.

4. The Enquiry depends for its success upon the co-operation of clinicians who take part, and therefore the maintenance of confidentiality and its educational and non-censorious nature.

5. The Enquiry encompasses selected events identified by clinicians, in respect of patients with one of the following conditions;

   (a)   Familial Adenomatous Polyposis.
   (b)   Cystic Fibrosis.
   (c)   Multiple Endocrine Neoplasia II.
   (d)   Down's Syndrome.
   (e)   Haemophilia.
   (f)   Thalassaemia
   (g)   Neural Tube Defect.

6. The Enquiry will concentrate on a manageably small number of clinical events relating to these disorders. It assesses what has been documented about the information and services offered to patients and their relatives, seeking:

   (a)   Documented evidence of appropriate counselling.
   (b)   Documented evidence of offer of relevant genetic services.
   (c)   Documented evidence of follow up, especially where potentially preventable late onset disorders are concerned.

7. Clinicians review their own records and are encouraged to involve their staff as a training process which will provide a framework of good practice for genetic disorders.

8. All hospitals within the Regional or Special Health Authorities of England, Wales and Northern Ireland are included. A variety of consultants from paediatrics, obstetrics, general surgery and other specialities are involved in addition to general practitioners.

APPENDIX 6 : Number of Counsellors compared with workload

Table 1 : 1991 centre 'workload' and number of counsellors

	Centre	Sickle cell disorder	Thalassaemia	Counsellors
Camberwell	1	645 (3)	? (0)	3
City & Hackney	2	330 (2)	18 (0)	3
Haringey	3	328 (2)	47 (0)	2
West Lambeth	4	360 (3)	3 (0)	0 / 1
Islington	5	252 (1)	95 (2)	1 / 1
Waltham Forest	6	300 (1)	6 (1)	1
Newham	7	248 (0)	17 (0)	1
Birmingham	8	190 (0)	50 (1)	3
Brent	9	200 (1)	6 (0)	4
Manchester	10	113 (2)	36 (0)	2
Bristol	11	67 (?)	5 (?)	0 / 1
Nottingham	12	48 (-)	5 (-)	1 / vacant
West Berks.	13	30 (0)	9 (1)	1
Leeds	14	17 (2)	17 (0)	2
Greenwich	15	31 (0)	- (0)	0 / 1
Coventry	16	30 (?)	? (?)	1
Wolverhampton	17	26 (-)	? (-)	1
South Glamorgan	18	17 (0)	8 (0)	2
Liverpool	19	3 (?)	2 (?)	0 / 1
South Derby	20	- (1)	- (0)	0 / 1
Total		3,233 (18)	324 (5)	28 / 6

Note : The details given above represent the perceived workload from the viewpoint of the relevant counsellors. These only include those in paid posts. In some cases the figures do not include "non-active" patients, that is ones not attending clinics. Figures for deaths are for the year 1991. The numbers given in brackets represent the numbers of deaths for SCD and thalasseamia that occured in 1991.

APPENDIX 7 : Summary of recommendations for management of major thalassaemia syndromes

Based on the "1992 Management protocol for the treatment of thalassaemia patients". (From the Thalassaemia International Federation, PO Box 8502, Nicosia, Cyprus).

AT PRESENTATION

It is important to distinguish thalassaemia major (over 90% of cases) from thalassaemia intermedia (less than 10% of cases). When the diagnosis is clearly thalassaemia major, maintenance transfusions should be started without delay. If there is reasonable suspicion of thalassaemia intermedia, i.e. the patient may survive in acceptable health without regular transfusion), it can be difficult to know what to do. On the one hand, the patient should be closely observed until the diagnosis becomes clear, but on the other delay in starting regular transfusion beyond the third birthday may allow the development of red cell antibodies that can make transfusion difficult if not impossible. Precise DNA genotyping may be very helpful in this differential diagnosis.

TRANSFUSION-DEPENDENT THALASSAEMIA

TRANSFUSION

In the absence of cardiomyopathy
1. Blood-type the patient completely
2. Vaccinate hepatitis B negative patients against hepatitis
3. Transfuse if the Hb remains consistently below 7g/dL (this does not apply if the patient is developing normally)
4. Keep the **mean** Hb between 12 and 12.5 g/dL
5. Give 10 –15 mL/kg of blood preparation in 2h
6. Do not raise the post-transfusion Hb above 15.5 g/dL
7. Choose a 2 – 4 week transfusion interval

In the presence of cardiomyopathy, or when the Hb is less than 5 g/dL:
8. Inject frusemide 1-2 mg/kg
9. Preferably use fresh blood
10. Do not transfuse more then 5 mL/kg of blood at one session
11. Do not transfuse faster than 2 mL/kg, maximum 4 h
12. Use short intertransfusion intervals

IRON CHELATION THERAPY

13. Desferrioxamine s.c. 20 – 50 mg/kg/day over 8 hr (average 40 mg/kg/day) plus 500mg-2g slowly i.v. with blood during transfusion.

14. In selected heavily iron-loaded subjects, give desferrioxamine i.v. 50 mg/kg/24h using short hospital admissions, or a Portacath. Higher doses may be considered for limited periods for patients with serious cardiac disease.

SPLENECTOMY

15. Is indicated when the blood consumption is more then 1.5 times "normal".
16. Give anti-pneumococcal vaccine 4 – 6 weeks **prior** to splenectomy.
17. Inform the patients and their family doctors of the increased risk of serious infections following splenectomy.
18. Give prophylactic penicillin and a platelet anti-aggregant when there is thrombocytosis in untransfused thalassaemia intermedia.
19. Infective episodes should be carefully observed and treated aggressively.

INVESTIGATIONS

Prior to treatment: study the case, and do complete red cell typing (ABO, Rhesus, Kell, Kidd and Duffy).

Before each transfusion: cross-match and test for a typical red cell antibodies in the serum. Record the date of transfusion, amount of blood transfused, and the pre-transfusion Hb.

After each transfusion: if feasible, measure the post-transfusion Hb (at 30 minutes or more after the end of the transfusion).

Every 3 months: record height and weight.

Every 6 months: ferritin estimation, evaluate growth. Measure Ca and phosphate, liver function tests, blood sugar, and thyroid function tests.

Every year: Evaluate growth and development. In children less than 12 years old, X-ray of hand and wrist. Calculate the transfusion indices. Evaluate iron balance.

Variable intervals: cardiac and endocrinological investigations according to the clinical state of the patient. Oral glucose tolerance test. In patients over 12 years, X-ray of knee to assess growth status.

THALASSAEMIA INTERMEDIA

Patients should be seen regularly (children at least every 3 months, adults every 6 months). Haemoglobin level, growth and spleen size should be monitored.

Numerous complications are possible and should be treated as they arise.

INVESTIGATIONS

At presentation: study the case. Include complete red cell typing (ABO, Rhesus, Kell, Kidd and Duffy).

Every 3 months: height, weight and spleen size.

Every 6 months: ferritin estimation, evaluate growth.

Every year: ferritin estimation
In children under 12 years, X-ray of hand and wrist.
Evaluate growth and development
Investigations according to the clinical state of the patient.

APPENDIX 8 : Psychological support

From the "1992 Management protocol for the treatment of thalassaemia patients". (Thalassaemia International Federation, PO Box 8503, Nicosia, Cyprus).

Although these recommendations have been prepared for patients with thalassaemia, many of them also apply to patients with SCD.

A WHO Working Group on Psychosocial Problems has evaluated recent experience and produced the following recommendations.

"Psychosocial support is and must remain an integral part of the total management of patients with haemoglobin disorders. It should be included in the service provided by the multidisciplinary team.

Overall responsibility for clinical care and co-ordination should rest with a single treating physician, who should remain the same for as long as possible, given the close relationship that develops between treating physician and patient. The team led by this physician should include a psychiatrist and/or psychologist and social worker. In order to emphasise the importance of psychosocial support, all members of the management team, especially nursing staff, should remain the same as long as possible and should have a thalassaemia/sickle cell oriented training. In particular, the mental health professionals should have some experience in management of patients with chronic diseases. The obligation of the team to reserve time and space for meetings with both patients and parents following each major visit to the treatment centre is of prime importance.

Families of children with inherited disorders such as the haemoglobin disorders, face an initial emotional crisis at the time of diagnosis. This can challenge the parental partnership and shift the whole balance of their family life. The family should be helped to accept the illness of the affected child and to understand its implications. They should be encouraged to understand and accept the need for orderly and continued surveillance and therapy. The parent should be helped to avoid overprotection of the affected child or children, in order to maintain the characteristics of a normally functioning family. They should therefore behave towards the affected child as far as possible in the same way as towards healthy siblings. In order to help the family in this, active participation in specific social programmes and interaction with other parents, self-help groups and patient associations can be very helpful.

The child with thalassaemia major or intermedia has to grow up on medical treatment and in continuous contact with health care professionals. The child may therefore appear (or feel) different from other children, and can have difficulty in establishing his or her body image. At an older age, particularly if puberty is delayed, the adolescent may feel dependent and experience problems in belonging to his peer group. The adolescent emotional crisis can be aggravated and the patient's development into adult life can become particularly complicated.

All patients should be helped to understand and accept their illness so that they can also accept the necessary treatment. They should be reassured that any complications which occur over the years do not necessarily mean a deterioration, and they should be encouraged to look to the future with optimism. It is therefore essential to encourage the patients' active participation in their own treatment programmes, and to help them to develop other interacting processes aimed at promoting their control of their own disease. Medical and psychosocial intervention should take account of the educational level and psychological strengths and weaknesses of individual patients, and help each according to his or her individual needs.

The integration of the child with a haemoglobin disorder into school constitutes a critical step in psychological development. The ultimate goal is the development of the child into an adult who can actively participate in society. In order to achieve this, the treatment team should contact the patients' schools and discuss the problems associated with their treatment, growth and development with the appropriate person. Schools should be encouraged to promote sensitisation of the teachers with respect to inherited diseases. The school staff should avoid allowing special privileges to children with haemoglobin disorders, except those which are medically indicated, in order to minimise the patients' dependency. The aim of everyone involved in the patients' care (family, physicians, psychiatrists, and teachers) must be to optimise integration of the patients into society. Efforts should concentrate on preparing them for the highest achievable level of work, rather than giving privileges which could lead to continued dependency."

PATIENTS' AND PARENTS' SUPPORT ASSOCIATIONS

Associations of parents and patients help families to feel less isolated, and let them know that they can depend on the help and comfort of others in the same situation. Even families who live too far away or are unwilling to participate directly, can benefit greatly from receiving Association literature. Through the Associations the families learn to see that their condition need not be completely overwhelming, and become more capable of coping with their own problems. Associations also facilitate the dialogue between patients and doctors which is such an important aspect of all chronic conditions, and so increase the patients' and the families' compliance with the treatment regime.

APPENDIX 9: Presentation of child in pain with Sickle Cell Disorder

an example of a protocol provided by the Hospital for Sick Children, Great Ormond Street

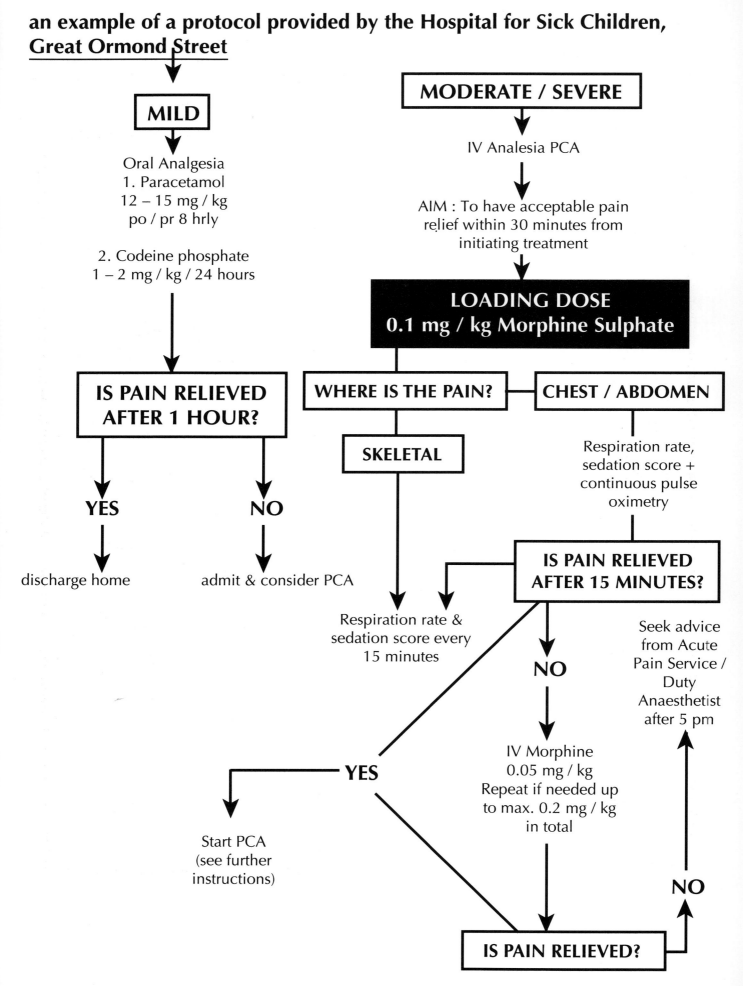

MILD

Oral Analgesia
1. Paracetamol
12 – 15 mg / kg
po / pr 8 hrly

2. Codeine phosphate
1 – 2 mg / kg / 24 hours

IS PAIN RELIEVED AFTER 1 HOUR?

YES

discharge home

NO

admit & consider PCA

MODERATE / SEVERE

IV Analesia PCA

AIM : To have acceptable pain relief within 30 minutes from initiating treatment

**LOADING DOSE
0.1 mg / kg Morphine Sulphate**

WHERE IS THE PAIN? — **CHEST / ABDOMEN**

SKELETAL

Respiration rate, sedation score + continuous pulse oximetry

Respiration rate & sedation score every 15 minutes

IS PAIN RELIEVED AFTER 15 MINUTES?

NO

IV Morphine
0.05 mg / kg
Repeat if needed up to max. 0.2 mg / kg in total

Seek advice from Acute Pain Service / Duty Anaesthetist after 5 pm

YES

Start PCA
(see further instructions)

IS PAIN RELIEVED?

NO

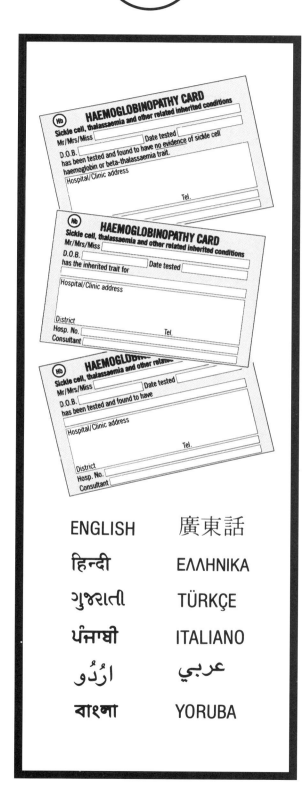

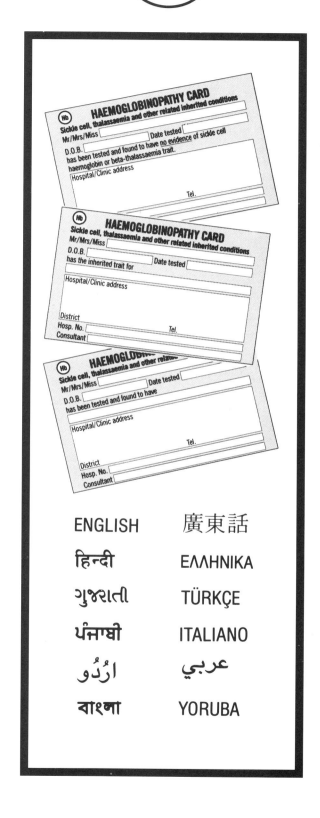

APPENDIX 11 : HAEMOGLOBINOPATHY TRIALS

Introduction

The usefulness of particular treatments and services for people with haemoglobinopathies was considered. One important method of evaluation is the randomised controlled trial (RCT), and the literature was reviewed to identify relevant RCTs.

It is important to recognise at the outset that RCTs are not the only useful method of evaluation. Their particular strength, however, is that their freedom from selection bias means that they can be used to detect 'moderate' benefits: that is, benefits that matter clinically but that may not be large enough to be spotted by clinicians.

Haemoglobinopathy RCTs published since 1984, were identified to (a) identify services of proven value (or of proven uselessness); (b) raise the question of how far the result of RCTs had been put into practice; (c) clarify R & D recommendations.

Methods and Results

Medline on Silverplatter was searched from 1983 to September 1992 inclusive. The search strategy was: 1) Random allocation (MeSH term); 2) Random (text word); 3) Clinical and Trial (text words); 4) Prospective or Prospectively (text words); 5) Double and Blind (text words) 6) Double Blind Method (MeSH term) 7) 1 or 2 3 or 4 5 or 6 8) Sickle cell anaemia (MeSH term) 9) Thalassaemia (MeSH term) 10) 7 and (8 or 9).

This search produced a list of 'probable' RCTs, the abstracts of which were then read to see if allocation to treatments was by random (or 'quasi-random': e.g. alternate) allocation. Copies of the papers were obtained for those studies where the abstract did not clearly specify the method of allocation.

This process produced a list of 29 trials that was circulated to members of the working group for comments and additions. This process identified one further randomised trial.

The 30 trials identified are listed, in alphabetical order of first author, on the attached sheet. This list is probably an underestimate of the true number of trials in the field, since (a) Medline was not searched for the years before 1983 and (b) it is known that Medline searches can miss up to 50% of trials in an area.

LIST OF TRIALS (ALPHABETICAL BY AUTHOR)

Baum KF, MacFarlane DE, Maude GH, Serjeant GR. Topical antibiotics in chronic sickle cell leg ulcers. Trans R Soc Trop Med Hyg 1987, 81(5): 847–9.

Benjamin LJ, Berkowitz LR, Orringer E, Mankad VN, Prasad AS, Lewkow LM, Chillar RK, Peterson CM. A collaborative, double-blind randomised study of cetiedil citrate in sickle cell crisis. Blood 1986; 67(5): 1442–7.

Billett HH, Kaul DK, Connel MM, Fabry ME, Nagel RL. Pentoxifylline (Trental) has no significant effect on laboratory parameters in sickle cell disease. Nouv Rev Fr Hematol 1989, 31(6): 403-7.

Cabannes R, Lonsdorfer J, Castaigne JP, Ondo A, Plassard A, Zohoun I. Clinical and biological double-blind-study of ticlopidine in preventive treatment of sickle-cell disease crises. Agents Actions Suppl 1984; 15: 199–212.

Chintu C, Gupta K, Osborne C, Masona JM. Clinical trial of the protective role of polyvalent pneumococcal vaccine in sickle cell anaemia patients in Zambia. Med J Zambia 1983; 17(3): 73–6.

Condon P, Jampol LM, Farber MD, Rabb M, Serjeant G. A randomized clinical trial of feeder vessel photocoagulation of proliferative sickle cell retinopathy. II. Update and analysis of risk factors. Ophthalmology 1984; 91(12): 1496–8.

Farber MD, Jampol LM, Fox P, Moriarty BJ, Acheson RW, Rabb MF, Serjeant GR. A randomized clinical trial of scatter photocoagulation of proliferative sickle cell retionpathy. Arch Ophthalmol 1991; 109(3): 363–7.

Gaston MH, Verter JI, Woods G, Pegelow C, Kelleher J, Presbury G, Zarkowsky H, Vichinsky E, Iyer R, Lobel JS, et al. Prophylaxis with oral penicillin in children with sickle cell anemia. A randomized trial. N Engl J Med 1986, 314(25): 1593–9.

Gonzalez ER, Bahal N, Hansen LA, Ware D, Bull DS, Ornato JP, Lehman ME. Intermittent injection vs patient-controlled analgesia for sickle cell crisis pain. Comparison in patients in the emergency department. Arch Intern Med 1991; 151(7): 1373–8.

Gonzalez ER, Ornato JP, Ware D, Bull D, Evens RP. Comparison of intramuscular analgesic activity of butorphanol and morphine in patients with sickle cell disease CM: Comment in: Ann Emerg Med 1989 May; 18(5): 603–5 Ann Emerg Med 1988; 17(8): 788–91.

Greenberg J, Ohene, Frempong K, Halus J, Way C, Schwartz E. Trial of low doses of aspirin as prophylaxis in sickle cell disease. J Pediatr 1983; 102(5): 781–4.

Jacobson MS, Gagliano DA, Cohen SB, Rabb MF, Jampol LM, Farber MD, Goldberg MF. A randomized clinical trial of feeder vessel photocoagulation of sickle cell retinopathy. A long-term follow-up. Ophthalmology 1991; 98(5): 581–5.

Jampol LM, Condon P, Farber M, Rabb M, Ford S, Serjeant G. A randomized clinical trial of feeder vessel photocoagulation of proliferative sickle cell retionpathy. I. Preliminary results. Ophthalmology 1983; 90(5): 540–5.

John AB, Ramlal A, Jackson H, Maude GH, Sharma AW, Serjeant GR. Prevention of pneumococcal infection in children with homozygous sickle cell disease. Br Med J Clin Res 1984; 288 (6430): 1567–70

Koshy M, Burd L, Dorn L, Huff G. Frequency of pain crisis during pregnancy. Prog Clin Biol Res 1987; 240: 305–11.

Koshy M, Burd L, Wallace D, Moawad A, Baron J. Prophylactic red-cell transfusions in pregnant patients with sickle cell disease. A randomized cooperative study CM: Comment in: N Engl J Med 1989 May 11; 320(19): 1286–7 N Engl J Med 1988; 319(22): 1447–52.

Manrique RV. Placebo controlled double-blind study of pentoxifylline in sickle cell disease patients. J Med 1987; 18(5–6): 277–91.

Marcus RE, Wonke B, Bantock HM, Thomas MJ, Parry ES, Taite H, Huehns ER. A prospective trial of young red cells in 48 patients with transfusion-dependent thalassaemia. Br J Haematol 1985; 60(1): 153–9.

Modell B, Letsky EA, Flynn DM, Peto R, Weatherall DJ. Survival and desferrioxamine in thalassaemia major. Br Med J Clin Res Ed 1982; 284(6322): 1081–4.

Olivieri NF, Koren G, St, Louis P, Freedman MH, McClelland RA, Templeton DM. Studies of the oral chelator 1, 2-dimethyl-3-hydroxypyrid-4-one in thalassemia patients. Semin Hematol 1990; 27(2): 101–4.

Olivieri NF, Templeton DM, Koren G, Chung D, Hermann C, Freeman MH, McClelland RA. Evaluation of the oral iron chelator L1, 2 dimethyl-3-hydroxypyrid-4-one (L1) in iron-loaded patients. Ann N Y Acad Sci 1990; 612: 369–77.

Pichard E, Duflo B, Coulibaly S, Mariko B, Mosempes JL, Traore HA, Diallo AD. [Effectiveness of treatment during osteoarticular pain crises in drepanocytosis; based on the example of pentoxifylline] TO: Evaluation de l'efficacite des traitements au cours des crises douloureuses osteo-articulaires de la drepanocytose: exemple de la pentoxifylline. Bull Soc Pathol Exot Filiales 1987; 80(5): 834–40.

Prasad AS, Cossack ZT. Zinc in sickle cell disease. Trans Assoc Am Physicians.1983; 96: 246–51.

Rabb LM, Grandison Y, Mason K, Hayes RJ, Serjeant B, Serjeant GR. A trial of folate supplementation in children with homozygous sickle cell disease. Br J Haematol 1983; 54(4): 589–94.

Rigau, Perez JG, Overturf GD, Chan LS, Weiss J, Powars D. Reactions to booster pneumococcal vaccination in patients with sickle cell disease. Pediatr Infect Dis 1983; 2(3): 199–202.

Semple MJ, Al, Hasani SF, Kioy P, Savidge GF. A double-blind trial of ticlopidine in sickle cell disease. Thromb Haemost 1984: 51(3): 303–6.

Serjeant GR, de Ceulaer K, Maude GH. Stilboestrol and stuttering priapism in homozygous sickle-cell disease. Lancet 1985; 2(8467): 1274–6.

Teuscher T, Von, Der, Ahe CW, Baillod P, Holzer B. Double-blind randomised clinical trial of pentoxiphyllin in vaso-occlusive sickle cell crisis. Trop Geogr Med 1989; 41(4): 320–5.

Wang WC, George SL, Wilimas JA. Transcutaneous electrical nerve stimulation treatment of sickle cell pain crises. Acta Haematol Basel 1988; 80(2): 99–102.

Zago MA, Costa FF, Ismael SJ, Tone LG, Bottura C. Treatment of sickle cell diseases with aspirin. Acta Haematol Basel 1984; 72(1): 61–4.

Authors (year)	Study group	No. in trial	Intervention/Control	Outcomes
Anti-pneumococcal prophylaxis				
Chintu et al (1983) [1,3]	People with sickle cell disease aged over 2 years and over	189	Polyvalent pneumococcal vaccine	Pneumococcal infection
Rigau Perez et al (1983) [2]	People with sickle cell disease	32	Booster pneumococcal vaccination/Placebo	Adverse reactions
John et al (1984) [2]	children aged 6 months to 3 years	242	Penicillin and pneumococcal immunisation/Placebo	pneumococcal infections
Gaston et al (1986)	Children with sickle cell anaemia under 3 years old	125	Oral penicillin/Placebo	Pneumococcal infection
Eyes: treatment				
Jampol et al (1983)	People with sickle proliferative retinopathy	167 eyes	Feeder vessel photocoagulation	Vitreous haemorrhage and visual acuity
Condon et al (1984)	People with proliferative sickle retinopathy	?	Feeder vessel photocoagulation	Visual acuity and vitreous heamorrhage
Farber et al (1991)	People with proliferative sickle retinopathy	174 eyes	Argon laser scatter photocoagulation therapy	Vitreous haemorrhage, visual acuity
Jacobson et al (1991)	People with proliferative sickle retinopathy	45 eyes	Feeder vessel photocoagulation	Vitreous haemorrhage and visual acuity

Authors (year)	Study group	No. in trial	Intervention/Control	Outcomes
Other				
Prasad et al (1983) [2]	14–19 year olds with sickle cell anaemia with retarded growth	?	Zinc	Height and weight
Rabb et al (1983) [2,5]	Children with HbSS, aged 6 months to 4 years	117	Folic acid supplements/Placebo	Haematological and clinical measures and growth
Serjeant et al (1985)	Men with HbSS with stuttering attacks of priapism	11	Stilboestrol/Placebo	Prevention of attacks
Baum et al (1987)	People with HbSS with chronic leg ulcers	30	Topical antibiotics	Ulcer size
Koshy et al (1988)	Pregnant women with sickle cell anaemia	72	Prophylactic red cell transfusions/therapeutic	Perinatal outcomes, including mortality
Thalassaemia				
Modell et al (1982)	People with homozygous beta-thalassaemia	?	Desferrioxamine	Survival
Marcus et at (1985)	Patients with transfusion-dependant thalassaemia major	48	Young red blood cells/Whole blood	Benefits and risks of transfusion
Olivieri et al (1990) [1]	"Thalassaemia patients"	?	Oral iron chelator (L1)	?
Olivieri et al (1990) [1]	"Iron-loaded patients"	?	Oral iron chelator (L1)	?

NOTES:
All studies were assessed for whether patients were randomised. They were all RCTs, except for those labelled [3,4] or [5]
[1] No abstract, so looked for original paper
[2] Uncertain from abstract, so looked for original paper
[3] From looking at paper, not clear if randomised
[4] From looking at paper, probably randomised crossover study
[5] From looking at paper, quasi-randomised (double blind with alternate allocation)

Authors (year)	Study group	No. in trial	Intervention/Control	Outcomes
Painful crises: prevention				
Greenberg et al (1983) [2,3,4]	children with sickle hemoglobinopathies	49	Aspirin/placebo	Frequency and severity of crises
Cabannes R, et al (1984) [1]	?	?	Ticlopidine	?
Semple et al (1984)	People with sickle cell disease	9	Ticlopidine/Placebo	Platelet studies and painful crises
Zago et al (1984) [2]	People with sickle cell disease	29	Aspirin/Placebo	Painful crises, infections, laboratory measures
Koshy et al (1987) [1]	Pregnant women	?	?	?
Manrique (1987)	People with sickle cell disease	60	Pentoxifylline/Placebo	Prevention of painful crises, haematological measures
Painful crises: treatment				
Benjamin et al (1966)	People with sickle cell disease with painful vasoocclusive crises	67	Cetiedil/placebo	Extent and duration of pain
Pichard et al (1987) [2]	People with sickle cell disease with painful crises	20	Pentoxifylline/Placebo	Intensity and duration of crisis
Gonzalez et al (1988)	People with sickle cell crises	18	Butorphanol/Morphine	Pain relief and adverse effects
Wang et al (1988)	People with painful sickle cell crisis	20 crises	Transcutaneous electrical nerve stimulation/Placebo	Pain ratings and analgesic requirements
Billett et al (1989)	People with painful sickle cell crises	16	Pentoxifylline/Placebo	Laboratory measures
Teuscher et al (1989) [1]	People with sickle cell disease with vaso-occlusive sickle cell crisis	?	Pentoxifylline	?
Gonzalez et al (1991)	People with sickle cell crisis in the emergency department	20	Intermittent IV analgesia/Patient Controlled Analgesia	Pain and alertness

NHS Management Executive

To: Regional General Managers
   District General Managers
   Unit General Managers
   General Managers of FHSAs
   General Managers of the Postgraduate SHAs

Copies to:
   Regional Directors of Public Health
   Regional Nursing Officers

PROFESSIONAL ADVICE FOR PURCHASERS: A DHA PROJECT DISCUSSION PAPER

1. Duncan Nichol wrote to you on 6 December last (EL(90)221) to reiterate the importance for both purchasers and providers of involving professional staff at all stages of drawing up contracts.

2. I now enclose a discussion paper produced by the NHS Management Executive's DHA project which considers the broader question of how DHAs as purchasers will in future have access to professional advice.

3. The paper describes how DHAs' current arrangements might evolve to reflect and accommodate the separation of the purchaser and provider functions. It follows discussions with managers and professionals in a number of health authorities, with those DHAs and RHAs working within the project, and with professional representatives within the Department. It takes account of the comments of the Joint Consultants Committee, the General Medical Services Committee and the Public Health Medicine Consultative Committee.

4. The paper's emphasis is on balance and continuity, and the need for new arrangements to evolve gradually. Discussions suggested that in future purchasers will require two broad types of professional advice, and the paper addresses both of these:

* <u>from providers with whom the purchaser has a contract</u> : the paper builds on the messages contained in EL(90)221 and the DHA project paper, <u>Starting Specifications</u> (EL(90)161).

* <u>independent advice</u> : for purchasers to have access to advice from professionals independent of any contractual interest with the particular District concerned.

The paper is aimed at helping DHAs develop their own local arrangements for professional advice.

5. I should be grateful if you would bring this letter and the discussion paper to the attention of your senior medical, nursing and other professional staff. The paper is not copyright and maybe freely reproduced. I am sending copies to the Joint Consultants Committee, the General Medical Services Committee, the Public Health Medicine Consultative Committee, the nursing professional organisations, professional organisations for therapists, and the Royal Pharmaceutical Society of Great Britain.

6. If you have any comments, please contact Hilary Symes at room G14A Richmond House, 79 Whitehall, London SW1A 2NS
Tel:071-210-5259; Fax:071-210-5523.

PETER GRIFFITHS
DEPUTY CHIEF EXECUTIVE
NHS MANAGEMENT EXECUTIVE

This letter will be cancelled on 31 August 1991

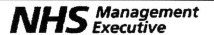

To: Regional General Managers
District General Managers
Unit General Managers
General Managers of FHSAs
SHA General Managers
General Managers of the Post Graduate SHAs
Regional GP Fundholding lead offices
                    (for information to GPFHs)

Department of Health
Richmond House
79 Whitehall
London SW1A 2NS
Telephone 071-210 3000

EL(93)60
2 July 1993

Dear Colleague,

Medical advice to purchasers

1. Health authorities need a range of professional and other advice if they are to discharge their purchasing role effectively.

2. The NHSME has been discussing with representatives of the medical professions how health authorities might secure sound medical advice.

3. The attached guidance has been prepared on the basis of these discussions and consultation with regions.

4. It is clear that the need for medical advice by health authorities arises at various stages in the purchasing process. This calls for a flexible approach which complements formal structures with local mechanisms suited to local needs. The guidance does *not*, therefore, prescribe how medical advice should be secured. It does, however, identify a number of key principles which *must* underpin the development of local medical advisory arrangements.

5. **Key action points**

DHAs and FHSAs should:

*   develop arrangements for securing sound medical advice which reflect the broad principles outlined in this paper; and

*   ensure that local clinicians know what mechanisms exist and that they have a defined access (eg through the Director of Public Health) to the purchasing process.

Regions should:

*   consider the scope for strengthening arrangements for securing external advice for purchasers; and

*   ensure that DHAs and FHSAs develop arrangements in line with paragraph 6.

6. The NHSME will monitor progress through the review process.

7. Enquiries about this guidance shuld be addressed to Helen Coley, room 4N34A, Quarry House, Quarry Hill, Leeds LS2 7UE   Telephone: 0532 545245.

Yours sincerely,

Alan Langlands
Deputy Chief Executive
NHS Management Executive

Graham Winyard
Director of Health Care
NHS Management Executive

This letter but not the attached guidance will be cancelled on 1 July 1994.

Medical Advice
for
Purchasers

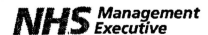

Medical advice for purchasers

1. This guidance draws on discussions with the medical profession nationally and on consultation with RHAs to:

i. reinforce the importance of sound medical advice for health authorities; and

ii. highlight key principles which should guide the development of medical advisory arrangements.

Background

2. Guidance on the need to involve professional staff in drawing up NHS contracts was set out in EL(90)221. The NHSME's discussion paper, "Professional Advice to Purchasers", issued in February 1991, outlined emerging ideas about how health authorities might secure access to professional advice. More recent guidance, EL(93)10 "Managing Activity and Change through Contracts", requires health authorities and provider managers to ensure that the terms of contracts, purchasing specifications, schedules of service and agreed activity levels are understood and agreed with clinicians and other professional staff.

3. This guidance focuses on medical advice. It should be noted, however, that a range of professional and other advice is needed by DHAs and FHSAs in order to discharge their roles effectively. The Priorities and Planning Guidance for 1993/94 (EL(92)47) requires health authorities to establish close links with local authorities, education and research bodies, providers and other local agencies including CHCs, voluntary organisations and the wider public. The contribution nursing can make to purchasing was explained in EL(93)36 issued in April 1993.

The need for medical advice

4. Medical advice needs to be taken into account at various stages in the purchasing process, particularly in:

*   **the assessment of health needs and development of health targets:** Directors of Public Health have a central role here because of their particular expertise to assess the health needs of the local population and as a focus for securing specialist advice from other sources. Medical advice is important in implementing the Health of the Nation strategy locally, in developing local health targets and linking these to contracts;

*   **determining priorities for health and targeting of resources:** medical advice should inform the initial identification of priority areas for evaluation, the appraisal of options for tackling health problems, the choice between competing priorities, and the subsequent development of purchasing plans and service specifications. Medical opinion about the relative effectiveness and cost-effectiveness of interventions and about developments in clinical practice is important in establishing the scope for trade-offs between different possible service changes (eg, between and within specialties, between and within client groups, between different treatments for the same condition, between secondary and primary care and between possible locations of care);

- **the negotiation and monitoring of contracts:** medical advice will be needed in defining clinical standards and outcome measures in contracts, in ensuring that contracts reflect GP referral patterns, and in assessing the workload and service implications of any proposed changes. Clinician involvement in the contracting process also enables more effective monitoring of contracts (eg, by making provider clinicians aware of contract activity thresholds and the action to take if these are reached, and by enabling GPs to alert health authorities if contract standards are not being met);

- **the handling of ECRs:** as stated in current guidance on ECRs, EL(92)60, the responsibility for handling ECRs must be shared between clinicians and purchasers and the process is most effective where purchasers have established close working relationships with the clinicians making the referrals;

- **the development of longer term health strategies:** the Priorities and Planning Guidance for 1993/94 requires DHAs to develop clear health strategies to provide at least a five year context for annual purchasing plans. Medical advice will be needed in developing these strategies, particularly to establish local health improvement targets, to take account of changes in clinical practice and medical technologies which are underway, or likely in the future, and to identify areas for research and development.

The need to develop medical advisory machinery

5.   Health authorities are required to recognise formally established Advisory Committees. Consultation with RHAs indicates that existing advisory frameworks continue to be widely used by purchasers to secure medical advice. Increasingly, however, these frameworks are being adapted, or new ones are being set up alongside them. The need for a changed approach to securing medical advice stems from:

- **the changing role of DHAs:** the separation of purchaser and provider functions, and the potential for flexibility as to where contracts are placed, makes it inappropriate for DHAs to rely exclusively on advice from local provider clinicians;

- **the need to strengthen GP involvement in purchasing:** to improve the balance between hospital and primary/ community services, and to make better use of GPs' as representatives of consumer views;

- **the re-configuration of health authorities:** local advisory arrangements need to be reviewed in the light of DHA mergers and the development of purchasing consortia;

- **the need for flexibility:** increasingly, purchasers require advice that is task-orientated and based on the particular experience, skills and knowledge of individuals rather than who they represent. This suggests a need for improved informal networking between Directors of Public Health, GPs, and consultants to complement formal "committee style" machinery;

- **the need for broad-based advice:** to reflect the increasing focus on people and their health rather than the management of services.

Key principles

6.   Consultations with RHAs have reinforced the NHSME's view that further central prescription about medical advisory arrangements would be inappropriate. It is vital, however, that arrangements for securing medical advice are robust, widely understood locally and that they command the confidence of health authorities and clinicians alike. Although local advisory arrangements should be tailored to local requirements, a number of common principles should be observed. These principles are:

- **broad-based involvement of GPs:** a number of approaches are being developed to involve GPs in purchasing, including GP fund-holding, locality purchasing, practice sensitive purchasing (based on the notional allocation of funds to practices), GP forums, advice from LMCs, surveys of GPs, regular practice visits, LMC representatives in contract teams, FHSA medical advisors, and GP representation on purchasing teams. There is unlikely to be a single right approach for any locality. The key aim should be to ensure that all GPs have the opportunity to contribute to the on-going cycle of purchasing activity (see paragraph 4 above). As part of this, GPs should be given regular feedback (eg through newsletters) about purchasing developments and how their views are being addressed.

- **direct relationships with provider clinicians:** direct purchaser dialogue with clinicians is *not* a substitute for discussions with provider managers but is essential if clinicians are to inform, understand and be committed to the terms of contracts. Each purchaser will need to establish with their providers (and their clinicians) the extent to which this should be done in a formal way or on a flexible basis. Approaches being developed include structured dialogue with clinical directorates, formal speciality and sub-specialty contract negotiations, formal discussions with local audit groups and informal discussions with individual clinicians (eg for ad hoc advice on specialist issues).

- **shared advisory arrangement between primary and secondary care clinicians:** there must be a forum for exchange of views between primary and secondary care clinicians. District Medical Advisory Committees have traditionally served this purpose. Purchasers will wish to consider the scope for strengthening existing opportunities for clinician-to-clinician dialogue and the need for multi-disciplinary fora. The options purchasers might consider include: joint DHA/FHSA advisory arrangements; joint GP, consultant and provider management advisory groups; multi-disciplinary groups to provide advice on wider health issues (eg including other professions, local agencies, and user and carer groups); and task-orientated clinical groups (eg to develop shared clinical protocols). The involvement of GP fund-holders in advisory fora should be encouraged and arrangements for securing advice should be made available to them;

- **access to external advice:** purchasers will need a broader medical perspective on certain issues than that available locally. Regions can offer this through:

  - the direct advice of the Regional director of Public Health;

  - access to regional networks, including Regional Medical Advisory Committees, Specialty Sub Committees, and Institutes of Public Health; and,

  - identifying and facilitating access to suitable professional national and international bodies.

A number of Regions are looking to strengthen arrangements for providing external advice and making these more sensitive to the needs of purchasers. The NHSME supports these developments.

Action

7.   DHAs and FHSAs should:

- develop arrangements for securing sound medical advice which reflect the broad principles and good practice outlined in this paper; and

- ensure that local clinicians know what mechanisms exist and that they have a defined access (eg through the Director of Public Health) to the purchasing process.

8.   Regions should:

- consider the scope for strengthening arrangements for securing external advice for purchasers; and

- ensure that DHAs and FHSAs develop arrangements in line with paragraph 6.

APPENDIX 13 : ANTI-SICKLING AGENTS – SUMMARY OF CURRENT STATUS

The approaches used to inhibit intravascular sickling may be broadly divided into (1) those inhibiting the gelation of haemoglobin S that occurs on deoxygenation, (2) those modifying the membrane rendering it less prone to sickling, and (3) those improving peripheral perfusion.

1. The first approach, inhibiting haemoglobin S gelation, has been the most promising. In the 1970's sodium cyanate was found to bond firmly to the haemoglobin molecule, carbamylating preferentially to the alpha chain, but also to a lesser extent the beta chain. There was a resultant increase in oxygen affinity and an anti-sickling effect. However, carbamylation also occurred in other enzyme systems and marked toxicity was observed. There was, furthermore, no objective evidence of decrease in painful crises despite improved haematological values.

   Substituted benzaldehydes were designed to bind preferentially to the oxy-conformation of haemoglobin at the alpha chain terminal amino region, thus increasing the oxygen affinity and reducing sickling. BW12C was found to increase oxygen affinity and cause a transient decrease in haemolysis in patients with sickle cell disorder. However, it was disadvantaged by a short half-life and an intravenous route of delivery. There have recently been short-term trials of an orally administered substituted benzaldehyde 589C80, which was found to be well absorbed orally, causing increased oxygen affinity and an anti-sickling effect. However at the initial dosages, adverse experiences were common and trials are at present underway on a modified regime hoping to allow longer term clinical studies to proceed.

   Other agents aimed to reduce polymerisation of deoxyhaemoglobin S by increasing the level of fetal haemoglobin. The cytotoxic drugs, hydroxyurea and 5-azacytidine were shown to increase fetal haemoglobin and cause a small reduction in haemolysis. These trials continue but as yet there is no convincing evidence of clinical benefit and the toxicity give concern for their long-term use.

2. A further approach was the use of membrane modifiers like phenothiazines, zinc and cetiedil. Cetiedil, an iminoester thought to inhibit calcium transport, seems the most promising. It was shown in two trials in the mid-1980s to cause a reduction in sickling, reducing the number of painful sites and duration of crises. However that trial work has not been further substantiated and the clinical role of this drug is uncertain.

3. The use of vasodilators like nifedipine, tolazoline, as well as anticoagulants to inhibit sickling, has met with little success in clinical trials.

SUMMARY

The need for anti-sickling agents to prevent or shorten sickle cell crises is an urgent one, especially in patients with severe disease. Promising candidates thus far are the substituted benzaldehyde (589C80), hydroxyurea and cetiedil but further toxicity and clinical studies will be required before general clinical use can be considered. A drug is unlikely to be available within five years.

ABBREVIATIONS

A & E   –   Accident and Emergency

ADA   –   Adenosine deaminase

BJA   –   British Journal of Anaesthetisia

BMJ   –   British Medical Journal

BMT   –   Bone marrow transplantation

CHS   –   Child Health Surveillance

DDPH   –   District director of public health

DNA   –   Deoxyribose nucleic acid

GP   –   General Practitioner

HLA   –   Human leucocyte antigen

IVF   –   In vitro fertilization

MCH   –   Mean cell haemoglobin

NEJM   –   New England Journal of Medicine

NSAID   –   Non-steroidal anti-inflammatory drug

OPCS   –   Office of population census and surveys

PUO   –   Pyrexia of unknown origin

SCD   –   Sickle Cell Disorder

SHPFH   –   Sickle trait with hereditary persistance of (high) fetal haemoglobin

SMAC   –   Standing medical advisory committee

GLOSSARY

Aplastic crisis — Infection typically by parvovirus B19 which leads to temporary shutdown of the marrow which produces red cells, white cells and platelets. In patients with sickle cell disorder the red cells have a decreased survival and patients are often already anaemic and so such infection can lead to very severe anaemia needing urgent blood transfusion.

Avascular hip necrosis — Repeated sickling within the hip leading to damage due to lack of blood supply. May need hip replacement in the long-term.

Carriers (heterozygote) (trait) — Individuals who have one normal haemoglobin gene producing normal haemoglobin (A) and one producing abnormal haemoglobin (HbS, HbC, B-thalassaemia, etc.)

Counselling (genetic) — Explaining to a person the transmission of genes within families generally and explaining to the individual if the individual is at risk of having a child with a major disorder.

Census — Questionnaire sent every ten years to all households in the UK to obtain information about the population regarding sex, age, number of children, ethnic background, etc.

Census ethnic groups — Categories of ethnic groups used in the census.

Controlled drugs — Drugs used for analgesia, usually opiates, which are controlled since they are liable to misuse and drug addiction – may be oral (taken by mouth) or parenteral (injection into the veins, muscle or under the skin).

Enuresis — Bed wetting

Entonox — A gas mixture of oxygen and nitrous oxide which is used to relieve moderate pain. Also used in labour wards.

Guthrie card — A card on which drops of blood from a recently born baby (within 7 days) are applied by a midwife to check for specific disorders – congenital hypothyroidism and phenylketonuria.

Haemoglobinopathy — Abnormality of haemoglobin.

Haemoglobinopathy card — A card given to people from ethnic groups at risk of haemoglobinopathy which states whether the person has the disorder, is a carrier or has normal haemoglobin genes.

Haemoglobin (Hb)	–	Red pigment present in the blood which carries oxygen.
	–	Hb A normal form of haemoglobin, HbS – sickle cell Haemoglobin.
Heterozygote	–	See carrier
Homozygote	–	Person with both genes of same type, e.g. HbSS – sickle cell disorder
Haemophilus influenzae	–	Infection which may cause severe pneumonia particularly if a person has no spleen or spleen is not working properly.
In vitro fertilisation	–	Fertilisation of an egg by a sperm outside the human body.
Iron chelation (desferrioxamine)	–	Removal of iron from the body to prevent deposition in the various organs of the body. Is necessary if a person has repeated blood transfusions. Drug currently used is desferrioxamine which is given either subcutaneously or intravenously.
Opiate / opiod	–	Drugs based on those derived from the opium poppy – see controlled drugs.
Painful crisis	–	Pain, typically in a bone, caused by red blood cells becoming sickled due to low oxygen.
Paraesthesiae	–	Tingling.
Parvovirus	–	See aplastic crisis.
Penicillin prophylaxis	–	Daily treatment with penicillin to prevent infection in children with sickle cell disorder with pneumococcus or haemophilus influenzae or salmonella.
Priapism	–	Persistent painful erection of the penis that requires decompression.
Primary health care	–	Care by a general practitioner in the community outside hospital.
Pulse Oximetry	–	Method of measuring amount of oxygen in the blood by placing a sensor onto the outside of the body (for example onto a finger) which does not require a blood sample to be taken.
Pump	–	A device which pumps a medicine such as desferrioxamine continuously into the body.

Register	–	An updated list of all individuals with a specific disorder.
Screening	–	Test performed to assess whether a person has a disorder or is at risk of a disorder.
	–	Antenatally – tests performed in pregnancy.
	–	Neonatal – of new babies.
	–	Non-directive – without trying to influence the person being counselled to make a particular decision.
	–	Opportunistic – as and when the need arises.
	–	Preconceptional – before a baby is conceived.
Self help groups	–	Groups of patients with a particular disorder or patients' relatives who meet to discuss common problems, to influence politicians and others, to raise awareness in the population.
Splenic sequestration	–	Accumulation of sickled red cells in the spleen. It is usually sudden and may cause severe anaemia and collapse.
Splenectomy	–	An operation to remove the spleen.
Thalassaemia major	–	The severe form of thalassaemia requiring regular blood transfusions if the affected person is to survive.
Thalassaemia intermedia	–	A less severe form of thalassaemia. Blood transfusion is only exceptionally needed.
Trait	–	See Carrier.

INDEX

Printed in the United Kingdom for HMSO.
Dd.0297614, C30, 12/93, 3397/5, 5673, 269434.